I CAN MAKE YOU
THIN

Also by Paul McKenna

I Can Make You Rich

Quit Smoking Today

Instant Confidence

I Can Make You Thin: 90-Day Success Journal

Change Your Life in Seven Days

I Can Mend Your Broken Heart
(with Hugh Willbourn)

The Hypnotic World of Paul McKenna

I CAN MAKE YOU

THIN ®

The Revolutionary System Used
by More Than 6 Million People

PAUL McKENNA, PhD

Edited by Michael Neill

STERLING
New York

STERLING
New York

An Imprint of Sterling Publishing
387 Park Avenue South
New York, NY 10016

ISBN 978-1-4027-6571-1 (hardcover)
ISBN 978-1-4027-7554-3 (paperback)

Distributed in Canada by Sterling Publishing
c/o Canadian Manda Group, 165 Dufferin Street
Toronto, Ontario, Canada M6K 3H6

For information about custom editions, special sales, and premium and
corporate purchases, please contact Sterling Special Sales at 800-805-5489 or
specialsales@sterlingpublishing.com.

Manufactured in the United States of America

2 4 6 8 10 9 7 5 3

www.sterlingpublishing.com

Warning

Do not listen to the CD while driving or operating heavy machinery, or if you suffer from certain neurological disorders including but not limited to epilepsy. If in doubt, consult your doctor.

The information and advice given in this book is designed to help you make informed decisions about your health. It is not intended as a substitute for any treatment that may have been prescribed by your doctor. If you suspect that you have a medical problem, we urge you to consult with your physician.

Contents

Preface

As a medical nutritionist for more than two decades, I have seen patients lose weight on any number of diet programs, then watched as they struggled to maintain their weight loss. The ability of overweight individuals to accept chronic food deprivation at levels as low as 400 calories a day for extended periods of time has never ceased to amaze me. Nor has the sad reality that most of them regain their hard-won losses. A significant number have undergone this process repeatedly.

Why couldn't obese individuals stay on a diet? Over the years, some patients told me they just couldn't stop themselves. Others said they ate mindlessly, often not knowing what they were eating. The common belief that eating is controllable has led us to expect people to "behave" or pay the price of public shame. But diets don't work: eating is not due to lack of willpower. Eating, ultimately, is under the control of the brain.

In our world, where food is freely available, maintaining weight loss by dieting requires a continuous conscious effort to eat less. Like our inability to resist sleep, our brains will override our minds and make us eat. This is in the nature of any living organism where the brain dictates behavior.

How can we alter this course? The answer lies not in the diet but in changing our response to signals from the brain. That is behavior modification. In this book are all the keys to accomplishing that which seems impossible: losing weight and keeping it off.

No fad diets are recommended here; rather, an approach to controlling the response to hunger and, even more importantly, a way of altering the appetitive drive by reducing the stress that dieting causes.

This is a revolutionary approach and it is the only approach that will be successful long term without the use of medication. I recommend that the reader keep an open mind and closely follow the expert advice given here. This approach requires work, but in persistence will lie victory for those who have long fought this battle.

—Ronald Ruden, MD, PhD
Lenox Hill Hospital, New York
Author of *The Craving Brain*

An Important Note from Paul McKenna

How would you like to eat whatever you want whenever you want and still lose weight?

I know that seems like an outrageous claim, and it's true.

The simple weight-loss system you are about to learn has created a revolution in England, where millions of people are using it. Now it's coming to America, where it is really needed.

We live in a culture of obsessive dieting and exercise addiction, yet recent studies have shown that two-thirds of the population of the United States is currently overweight. What's gone wrong?

A growing army of medical doctors has been compiling more and more evidence that proves what I've known for years:

Diets are the enemy of weight loss!

The overwhelming scientific evidence shows that diets work for less than 10 percent of the people who use them. The problem is that the vast majority of people who come off a diet end up putting on more weight than before they went on it. And diets are not just a symptom of the problem—they are a significant part of its cause. I am completely serious when I say that there is a better case for banning diets than banning smoking when we consider the health consequences to America.

I am on a mission to help the world lose weight and to make the process as easy as possible. My system is so simple you may find it difficult at first to believe how quickly it will work. That's because you have been brainwashed by the dieting industry to believe that weight loss is difficult, and it's not. If it's difficult, you're doing something wrong.

Here is all you need to do to begin using what millions of people agree is the simplest weight loss system in the world:

1. Read this book. It will take you approximately two hours.

2. Follow the instructions.

3. Use the hypnosis CD every day for two weeks.

4. Notice your eating patterns change and the weight drop off.

It's that simple!

Recently I met a lady who attended one of my seminars and lost a considerable amount of weight. She told me that she was angry. When I asked her why, she said it was because she had spent years torturing herself with diets and feeling like a failure. In fact, she'd added up all the money she'd spent on diets, weight-loss programs, and special foods, and it came to nearly twenty thousand dollars. If only she'd known how easy weight loss really is, she could have saved herself all that money and years of unnecessary stress.

Much of what I am about to say will fly in the face of what you've done in the past and what you think is "right." You've tried other methods of weight loss and they didn't work or they only worked temporarily.

No matter what you've tried before, it's time to do something radically different.

The exact same approach that I am about to share with you has helped millions of people to lose weight easily and feel significantly better about themselves. In fact, two independent research studies into the effectiveness of my system showed that what you are about to learn is seven times more effective than any diet.

Now it's your turn!

To your good health.

—Paul McKenna
Los Angeles, 2008

The Weight-Loss Hypnosis CD

Your mind is like a computer—it has its own software, which helps you to organize your thinking and behavior. Having worked with all sorts of people with different problems over many years, I have learned that almost all problems stem from the same cause: negative programs running in the unconscious mind.

This book comes with a powerful hypnosis CD that will fill your unconscious mind with positive willpower. While you become absorbed into a natural state of relaxation, I will reprogram your computer—your unconscious mind—so that you will change the way you think about food and feel better about yourself. I will give you suggestions that will help you to change your behavior, eat better, speed up your metabolism, and escape from the fixation with food.

It's best to listen to it when you have about a half hour where you can safely relax completely. As you listen to it regularly, you will reinforce all the changes you are making. In fact, it will make it much easier to stick to the golden rules I share with you in this book.

The latest research into the effectiveness of these and similar techniques has shown that listening to this CD over and over again, every day, will dramatically enhance your ability to lose weight. You don't have to believe it, only use it!

1.

Are You Ready for Something Completely Different?

This may well be the shortest book on losing weight you have ever read. But don't be fooled by its size. As I think you'll agree, thin is good, and it's what's inside that really matters.

I've worked hard to make this little book as concise as possible—so concise that you can probably finish the whole thing in less than a day. But what a day it will be!

During that time, you will not only discover what's been keeping you from the body you desire, but you'll also learn the simplest and most effective weight-loss system ever devised. It's a system that has helped people who felt as though they had failed at every diet in the world, or been overweight all their lives, as well as those people who just wanted to lose weight and feel great for life.

Whether your primary goal is to lose weight, lead a healthier lifestyle, feel really happy with your body, or just to be able to lose those last ten pounds, this system is exactly what you've been looking for!

I'll also reveal the truth about exercise and share with you some simple but powerful techniques to supercharge your metabolism, control your cravings, and let go of the emotional issues you used to stuff down with food. Finally, I'll teach you some of my favorite hypnosis techniques, which you can use to feel better now and in the future; you'll be able to put on the CD any time you want to reinforce the principles deep into your unconscious mind.

But don't take my word for it—just follow my instructions step by step and notice how your body, and life, begin to change for the better.

Learning the Secrets of Naturally Thin People

Throughout the book, I will share with you the secrets I have gleaned by studying naturally thin people. These are not the stick-figure models whose waiflike physiques come from eating disorders, drug addiction, and airbrushing, but rather those people in life who somehow seem to be able to eat whatever they want and stay slim.

By developing the eating habits of naturally thin people, you'll be able to eat anything you want, whenever you want, and still lose weight. Let's face it: you can have what you want, or you can have your reasons for not having it. So, if *absolutely anyone can lose weight with this system*, the only other question we need to ask is this:

Why aren't you thin yet?

There are three main patterns I have observed that keep people from living happily at their desired weight. As you read through the descriptions below, notice which of these apply to you. Then, when we begin reprogramming your mind in chapter 3, you will be able to apply just the right tools and begin to lose weight immediately . . .

Pattern One: Obsessive Dieting

I was browsing through some of the recent releases in the weight-loss section of my local bookstore. What I found astounding was that despite the fact that nearly all of them were filled with "forbidden food" lists, menus, and calorie guides, they each began with the words "This is NOT a diet."

Let's begin by getting one thing straight:

> **A diet is any system of eating that attempts to exert external control over what, where, when, or how much you eat.**

Dieting has gotten a bad name over the past few years, and there's a good reason for that—scientific research shows that more than 90 percent of people who attempt to lose weight by dieting fail.

Whenever somebody comes up to tell me about the weight they've lost on this great new diet, I ask them to come back and tell me about it in six months' time. If they are still happy about their weight and their diet in six months I am ready to listen. Unfortunately, I am still waiting for anybody to come back.

My theory? Too many diets, too few results. With over 25,000 diet books currently in print, many of which contain directly contradictory information, is it any wonder you find yourself as confused and misguided as the multi-billion-dollar weight-loss industry?

It's not just that diets don't work: many of them are an outright con. In fact, when I see celebrities who have "battled their weight problems" endorsing the latest fad diet, I don't know how they keep a straight face. In most instances, what they have actually done is tried a diet, lost weight, and then put the weight back on again a few months later. Then they simply tried another diet, lost weight, and promoted that one for a few months until the weight started piling back on.

In case you haven't picked up on the message here, it's this:

Forget about dieting. Forever. Diets are essentially training courses in how to get fat and feel like a failure.

The more diets people try and fail at, the more they convince themselves they will never be able to lose weight. What nobody tells you is that the real reason most weight-loss programs don't work has nothing to do with you—it's to do with human biology.

In his seminal study into human starvation during

the Second World War, biological researcher Ancel Keyes discovered that reducing people's diet to a state of semi-starvation produced symptoms of irritability, loss of endurance, and obsessive behavior around food, including but not limited to lying, hoarding, and stealing.

Even more telling, in the three-month period after the semi-starvation was ended and people could once again eat whatever they wanted, their obsession with food continued. Many people ate up to eight times as much food as they had done before the study began. (Does any of this sound familiar?)

That experiment, documented in the 1950s treatise *The Biology of Human Starvation*, is considered unreplicable. After all, to starve people purposely would be cruel and inhumane. But here's an interesting fact: the semi-starvation rations from the original study amounted to about 1,500 calories a day—more than is allowed in any number of the thousands of diets currently in vogue.

What all this goes to show is that depriving yourself of food is the worst possible way to lose weight. And if what you're doing isn't working, you need to do something different.

Pattern Two: Emotional Eating

I am convinced that after diets, emotional eating is the number-one cause of obesity in the world. Many times people eat because they are bored or lonely or miserable or tired, or any one of a hundred emotional reasons, none of which has anything to do with physical hunger. If you eat based on emotional hunger, your body will never feel satisfied by food. This is why many people think that they never feel full—they never get the signal to stop eating because they were never hungry for food in the first place.

Maybe you first put on weight following a trauma or difficult time in your life and you began to comfort-eat to help you through that time. Now, even though that stressful time is past, you have kept the dysfunctional habit of eating when you feel upset, lonely, or just bored. This habit stems from a fundamental misunderstanding of why we feel what we feel.

An emotion is a bit like someone knocking on your door to deliver a message. If the message is urgent it knocks loudly; if it's very urgent it knocks very loudly; if it is very urgent and you don't answer the door, it knocks louder and louder and louder until you open the door or it breaks it down. Either way, the emotion will continue to come up until it's done its job. As soon as you "open the door" by listening to the emotional message and taking appropriate action, the emotion will simply go away.

The good news is that with this new understanding, you don't have to be a victim anymore. While I will be sharing a number of powerful techniques in the chapter on emotional eating, one of my colleagues has achieved an extraordinary amount of success by simply making his clients put a giant question mark on their fridge. The question mark is there to remind them to stop before grabbing a snack and ask themselves this question:

Am I really hungry, or do I just want to change the way I feel?

If it turns out that what you actually want is a change in the way that you feel, no amount of food will work as well as applying the simple techniques in this book and on the hypnosis CD.

One Additional Thought

I am continually surprised at the number of women (and occasionally men) I work with who realize that their initial weight gain coincided with a traumatic incident from the past, ranging from episodes of sexual abuse to seemingly innocuous teasing leading to embarrassment in front of their peers.

While the techniques in this book and on the hypnosis CD will help, they are not intended as a substitute for professional guidance. If you suspect this could apply to you, ask your doctor to recommend an appropriate therapist.

Pattern Three: Faulty Programming

If you are overweight it's not your fault—it's the natural result of your current mental programming, and no diet, pill, shake, or how-to book can change that. The only way to lose weight and keep it off is to go to the unconscious mind and change your relationship with food forever.

So relax. You are not crazy, you are not broken, and

you are not a bad person. You have simply developed some very unproductive habits. The good news is that once you learn to reprogram your mind, it will be just as simple to develop new habits of thinking and acting that will guarantee your success.

You don't even have to believe that it will work. Just follow my instructions and you will not only lose weight but stop obsessing about food forever.

In just a few minutes, I'm going to share with you the four most important things you will ever learn about losing weight and keeping it off for life. But before we get started, I want you to stop for a moment and do the thought experiment on the opposite page.

The Power of Perspective

Go to near the end of your life. Imagine that it is many years from now and you decided *not* to follow my instructions and begin losing weight. Instead, you went on trying one diet after another, continuing to gain weight and lose your precious vitality year after year after year . . .

- What were the consequences of that decision on your health?

- What were the consequences on your relationships?

- What were the consequences on your sense of well-being?

- How do you feel in your body?

Now . . . take a few moments to imagine following this program and easily reaching and maintaining your target weight.

- How good does this feel?

- How much energy do you have?

- What are you able to do?

- What clothes are you able to wear?

- Who are you with? What are you doing?

- Exactly what will it be like when you have lived at your target weight for years and years?

Now . . . *stop!*

It's time to decide. If you want to hang on to your excuses and your excess weight, you may as well put the book down now.

But if you're ready finally to get that monkey off your back (and those inches off your waist), know that what you do from this moment onward is entirely up to you. So let's get started!

"Are You Ready for Something Completely Different?"

Q. I've tried lots of different ways to lose weight and none of them have worked. How is your system different?

In a fascinating study at the University of Hertfordshire, Professor Ben Fletcher achieved spectacular results by teaching people to respond to their "hunger pangs" by going out and doing something in the world—turning off the TV and going for a walk, speaking with a friend, or even going out to a movie. As a result of "doing something different" around food, their habits began to change. People naturally began to make healthier choices around food and exercise.

The reason nothing's worked before is you've done the same thing over and over again—you've systematically starved yourself by dieting. The only thing you've changed is the recipes. And the definition of insanity is doing the same thing and expecting a different result!

Q. What if I'm really overweight—can I still use this system or do I need to diet first?

This system is directly at odds with any and every diet you might try, because it's diets and the dieting mentality that were making and keeping you overweight in the first place!

At the risk of repeating myself, I'll say it one more time:

Anything or anyone who tries to tell you what, where, when, or how much to eat is teaching you to ignore your body—and if you're overweight, your body is trying to tell you it doesn't like being ignored!

I don't care how much you weigh, if you've been overweight all your life, or if all your family are overweight—as you use this system you will lose weight and feel more in control and better about yourself.

Q. How well does this work? I want to look like the models in magazines.

So do the models in the magazines. Most of the pictures you see on magazine covers have been digitally altered in order to make them striking so that you will buy the magazine. They are not representative of reality. Rather than compare yourself to something that doesn't exist, it's far better to compare yourself to yourself. Far too many women compare themselves with an airbrushed picture of an anorexic girl on a magazine cover and decide they aren't good enough as a human being. You are likely to feel significantly better if you ask yourself this question instead:

How much better am I getting?

Actually, I lived in New York for a number of years and had the opportunity to meet many of the world's most famous models. What struck me was that even though many of these women looked so incredibly beautiful, they were pretty miserable, which I suppose is understandable given that they're so hungry all the time! I realized that they spent all their time looking for flaws and rarely saw the perfection of who they already were.

As the great philosopher Goethe said, "It's not so important where we stand, but the direction in which we are moving." Human beings are usually at any time either getting better or worse. If you are getting better, excellent. If you are getting worse, then you know the direction in which you need to move.

Kate's Story

Kate Howlett

Lost 77 pounds

Before   **After**

Before starting the Paul McKenna weight-loss system, I had tried every sort of diet: fat counting, calorie counting, I even tried not eating until after five o'clock in the evening. I had finally given up. I was fat. It ran in my family. What could I do about it? Then a colleague told me she'd done the Paul McKenna system and she was feeling really good, so I thought I'd give it a try.

Once I started doing it, I was amazed how easy it

was to lose weight. I realized that this was not a diet, but a new way of looking at food. Now I enjoy my food, instead of spending all my time thinking about it and then wolfing it down thoughtlessly, like I used to. The only problem is in restaurants where the portions are too big and I have to explain that the food was good but just too much.

I still listen to the CD. It says I'll have more energy on waking up—and I do. I enjoy walking my son to school; I always used to take the car. One of my greatest pleasures now is shopping for clothes, which is something I used to dread.

Since doing the Paul McKenna system, I feel much more positive about life. In a way, the weight loss is just a bonus!

Kate lost 77 pounds over 12 months. Generally, people who used this program lost, on average, 1–2 pounds per week.

2

The Simplest Weight-Loss System in the World™

The "Secrets" of Naturally Thin People

Sometimes people ask me how I came up with this system. Was I ever overweight myself? Did I study physiology in college? Did I just conjure it up out of thin air?

The reality is, it's taken me more than twenty years to develop this system and refine it to the point that I can share it with you today in the pages of a book. Over that time, I compared the mindsets and strategies of chronically overweight people with those who seemed to be "naturally thin."

What I discovered is that there are no "naturally thin" people—it's just that some people were fortunate enough not to have been brainwashed by diets and the weight-loss industry into ignoring their bodies and blindly following the medical establishment, many of whom are funded by the very weight-loss industry they so heartily recommend.

Your body is smarter than any diet on earth, but with volumes of information all around us about how the "wrong" foods will adversely affect our health or make us put on weight, it can be difficult to see, hear, or feel what your body is telling you. That's why what I am about to explain to you is all you really need to change the way you eat forever.

The real secret of being naturally thin is simply to introduce four new habits into your life—four "golden rules" for deciding when to eat, what to eat, how to eat it, and how much of it to have. These small habits will make a huge difference in your life—four simple guiding principles that will help you to make the best food choices in any situation you may encounter . . .

GOLDEN RULE NUMBER 1

When you are hungry, EAT

How Starving Yourself Can Actually Make You Fat

Ever wonder what's inside a camel's hump? It's fat—stored fat. Camels store fat because they don't know how long they're going to go between meals. When you starve yourself by not eating when you're hungry, your body does the same thing. In fact, if you've been trying to lose weight for a while, your body is probably stuck in continual fat-storage mode. When you starve your body, it freaks out and goes into survival mode because it thinks there is a famine and stores fat in your cells, "just in case." Over time, your body begins to leach more fat from whatever foods you do eat. There may be only a few grams of fat in that diet lasagna, but if you're eating at "mealtimes" instead of when you're hungry, your body will do whatever it takes to grab on to that fat and put it where it can store it until later—generally your stomach if you're a man and your hips and thighs if you're a woman.

That's partly why thin people can eat a lot and not put on weight—they aren't starving themselves, so their bodies can either make use of or easily eliminate excess fat that comes from their food.

In addition, consistently overriding your body's natural call for food alters your metabolism. A faster metabolism burns more calories throughout the day, but when you stop yourself from eating when you're hungry, your metabolism slows down so your body can conserve energy. This leads to feelings of lethargy, which many people experience as a mild depression.

If all that wasn't enough, not eating when you're hungry sets up dysfunctional patterns of thinking in the unconscious mind in relation to food. This subtle tension around food sets up a powerful neurochemical change in the brain that leads to false hunger signals and patterns of craving and bingeing. The vicious cycle is in motion—the less you trust your body, the less trustworthy your body's messages become.

There is, however, some very good news:

All you need to do to reset your
body's innate wisdom is to eat whenever
you feel truly hungry.

True hunger is different than emotional hunger (which we will deal with in chapter 4). If you read the first golden rule and said to yourself, "But I'm hungry all the time!" or even "But I'm never hungry," chances are what you're experiencing is more emotional than physical. Fortunately, as soon as you begin to listen to your body, you will once again be able to recognize easily the subtle and not so subtle signs of true, authentic hunger.

The Hunger Scale

At this point I want to introduce you to an amazing tool that you can use to know exactly when to start eating and when to stop. I call it the hunger scale. The hunger scale goes from one, which is physically faint with hunger, to ten, which is stuffed to the point of nausea.

Take a few moments right now to look at the hunger scale on page 30 and tune in to your body. How hungry are you right now?

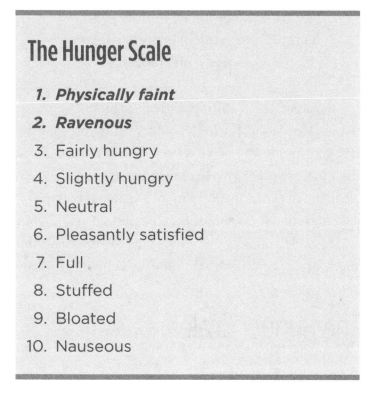

The Hunger Scale

1. *Physically faint*

2. *Ravenous*

3. Fairly hungry

4. Slightly hungry

5. Neutral

6. Pleasantly satisfied

7. Full

8. Stuffed

9. Bloated

10. Nauseous

Each person is different, but as a general rule you'll want to eat whenever you notice yourself between 3 and 4 on the scale—that is when you are fairly hungry, but before you become ravenous. If you wait until you get down to 1 or 2, your body will go into starvation mode and you'll probably wind up eating more than your body needs and storing the excess as fat.

Of course, if you have been a serial dieter you may be so used to overriding your body's signals that you may at times "forget to eat" until you're already ravenous. If you think this might be you, practice tuning in to your body once an hour and giving yourself a number from 1 to 10 until you begin to notice differences between the points on the scale.

The more you practice tuning in to your own hunger, the sooner you'll be able to recognize your body's subtle signals long before your stomach growls and your brain starts to get fuzzy.

GOLDEN RULE NUMBER 2

EAT WHAT YOU WANT, not what you think you should

Resistance Is Futile

In a fascinating experiment performed in the 1930s, scientists gave a group of toddlers unlimited twenty-four/seven access to a vast range of foods from ice cream to spinach, essentially allowing them to create their own diet over a period of thirty days based on their own sense of what they wanted to eat and when.

The result?

While they each chose different foods at different times, every single child in the study wound up eating what was considered to be a balanced diet over the course of the month.

Similarly, many women have had the experience of

unusual food cravings during pregnancy. The reason a pregnant woman will crave everything from ice cream to pickled onions is that her body is telling her exactly what it needs from moment to moment to "build a baby."

But as soon as you tell yourself not to eat certain foods (usually because you've been told they're bad for you), you upset the natural balance of your relationship to them. Rather than wanting it less, that "forbidden food" instantly becomes more attractive to you. The inner battle between your positive intention and your resistance to being controlled (even by yourself) can be exhausting. As you begin to make peace with food and learn to listen to the wisdom of your body, you experience freedom from the tension and guilt that come from *not* following your intuition.

This is why there are *no* forbidden foods in my system—you can eat anything you want any time you are hungry, providing you take the time to really, really enjoy it (see Golden Rule number 3!).

In fact, why not go one step further?

You may in the past have been on one diet or another that told you to empty your cupboards of any foods high in fat, sugar, carbohydrates, or whatever food you were being forbidden to eat.

My instructions for you are radically different.

Today, as soon as you finish reading this book, I want

you to go to your refrigerator and throw out any food that does not totally inspire you to eat it. Chuck the diet soda. Throw out the low-fat yogurts. Unless you absolutely love them, get rid of the sugar-free Popsicles. You'll know that you're done when there isn't a single thing in your fridge that you wouldn't be delighted to eat—and when you're next hungry, that's exactly what I'm asking you to do.

Care for a bit of pasta?

Go for it.

Cake and ice cream calling to you?

As long as you're actually hungry, enjoy, enjoy, enjoy.

From this day forward, nothing is off-limits to you. Ever.

And if you really want to say "NO" to something, say it to the purveyors of sugar-free low-carb cardboard-tasting crap.

GOLDEN RULE NUMBER 3

Eat CONSCIOUSLY and enjoy every mouthful

Conscious Eating

I've noticed a funny thing about people who are overweight. They spend all their time thinking about food—except when they're actually eating it. Then they go into a kind of "eating trance," where they shovel as much food into their mouths as fast as they can without actually chewing or tasting anything.

Strange as it may seem, there is a very good reason for that. Whenever we do something that is essential for our survival, like eating, breathing deeply, or making love, we release a "happy chemical" in our brains called serotonin.

People who are overweight often shovel food into their mouths as quickly as possible in order to get a serotonin high. Unfortunately, because they are eating unconsciously, they never notice the signal from their stomach that lets them know that they are full. So they keep on stuffing their faces, expanding their stomachs and putting on weight.

The problem is that even though they feel temporarily high from cramming in lots of food, they feel fat and guilty afterward. In fact, they feel so bad that they repeat the whole ritual of unconsciously stuffing themselves again in order to anesthetize the bad feelings they just created!

One of the unique features of my weight-loss program is this:

> *You can eat whatever you want,*
> *whenever you want, so long as you fully*
> *enjoy every single mouthful.*

I cannot emphasize this enough. I mean *really* enjoy it—savor the taste and enjoy the wonderful textures and sensations as you thoroughly chew each mouthful. Of course, in order to fully enjoy your food, you have to notice that you're eating it.

I remember seeing a friend of mine who had lost a ton of weight and looked amazing. When I asked her how she had done it, she told me that she had just returned from a luxury health resort in the Far East at a cost of two thousand dollars a day. When I asked about the basis of the weight-loss regime they had used, she explained that in the West, we eat far too quickly.

At the spa, they taught her to slow her eating speed and become more conscious of the process of smelling, tasting, and chewing her food. Each meal was like a meditation, and to help her to remember to do it, the spa assigned someone to sit opposite her during every meal and constantly remind her to slow down and savor each mouthful.

To put this to work for you, here is one simple thing you can do to help you enjoy each mouthful as a new and positive habit:

> ***For the next two weeks, slow your eating speed down to about a quarter of what it used to be and chew each mouthful thoroughly.***

It's very important to put your knife and fork down between every mouthful, so you can give your body time to notice what it's doing. Of course, if you're not using cutlery, take your fingers off your sandwich and put it down between each mouthful. When your mouth is empty, you can pick up where you left off.

In this way, you make every bite a conscious choice, eating your food like a gourmet and savoring every mouthful instead of shoveling it in on automatic like a barnyard animal.

The Importance of Eliminating Distractions

Of course, eating consciously does not only mean eating slowly. Until you really get the hang of this system, it means concentrating on your food and nothing else. A recent study conducted in Switzerland showed that when people were blindfolded, they ate 25 percent less than when they could see—in other words, when they weren't looking at the food but were instead totally concentrating on the taste and texture, they actually ate less.

This corresponds with what I've noticed at my weight-loss seminars. After lunch, people will often report that their food tasted amazing, because for the first time in ages they were eating slowly and consciously enough to actually taste it and notice the feeling of being full.

Professor Brian Wansink, author of the amazing book *Mindless Eating*, has conducted some extraordinary experiments that show conclusively that when we are distracted during the process of eating, we not only don't notice what we are eating, we eat substantially more of it.

You can probably remember for yourself a time when you were eating popcorn, nuts, or chips while watching a film or a football game. By the time you "woke up" and came to your senses, the entire bowl, bag, or box was empty, no matter how hungry you were when you started.

Since studies show that a whopping 91 percent of people eat in front of the television, a powerful way to begin disrupting your old unconscious habits is simply to stop eating while reading, chatting on the phone, or watching the TV. By eliminating as many distractions as possible while you eat, at least when you are first learning this system, you will find it considerably easier to notice and apply the fourth golden rule . . .

GOLDEN RULE NUMBER 4

When you think you are full, STOP eating

Your Inner Thermostat

I remember as a kid using my mother's electric kettle to steam open an envelope. In order to keep the steam rising, I had to hold the "on" switch down long after the kettle had boiled. Of course, kettles aren't designed to be used that way, and soon the metal thermostat inside the kettle became bent and stopped working properly.

Fortunately, it was quite easy to fix. All I had to do was go inside and bend the thermostat back into place. Immediately, the kettle began working perfectly again.

The natural design of the human body is to eat when we're hungry and stop when we're satisfied, but many of us are conditioned to eat until we think we're full—or even worse, until whatever food we put on our plate is gone.

To lose weight effortlessly and keep it off, you must begin working with your body and not against it. To get slim and stay slim we need to resensitize ourselves to our "inner thermostat" so we can stop eating when we are full and feel good for the rest of the day.

In reality, when you've eaten enough, your stomach sends a signal—a sensation that says, "I'm satisfied—that's enough."

Although studies have shown that it can take up to twenty minutes for that signal to reach your brain, when you slow down your eating speed and eat more consciously, it becomes easier and easier to notice this signal as soon as it's sent. Most people experience it as a gentle, clear, satisfied sensation in their solar plexus (the area below your rib cage but above your stomach).

Even if you miss this warm feeling of satisfaction when it first occurs, there's another way to know that your stomach is full. As soon as you've had enough to eat, you'll notice that each subsequent bite of food becomes a little less enjoyable than the one before. The more you pay attention to this phenomenon, the more obvious it becomes.

Since continuing to eat after this satisfied feeling begins to emanate from your solar plexus produces distinct and ever increasing sensations of discomfort, it is important that as soon as you begin to notice this discomfort, you stop eating immediately, no matter how much or how little food is left on your plate.

When I teach this in my seminars, there is invariably one person who starts to panic and say, "But what if I'm hungry again ten minutes later?"

The answer is very simple: if you're hungry, *eat*. However, you must *eat what you actually want*, not what you think you should; eat *consciously* and enjoy every mouthful, and then once again when you even suspect you are full, *stop*.

Revisiting the Hunger Scale

If you have ever been a serial dieter, you may be so used to overriding your body's signals that you keep eating until you're full or even stuffed before noticing it's time to stop. I cannot overemphasize what a useful tool the hunger scale will be for you. Becoming aware of what your body needs and wants is like a muscle—the more you use your awareness, the stronger it gets. When it comes to knowing when enough is enough, you'll want to stop eating at around 6 or 7 on the hunger scale— when you are feeling pleasantly satisfied or full but not yet stuffed or bloated. Simply *never* live in the extreme areas of the hunger scale ever again.

The Hunger Scale

1. ***Physically faint***
2. ***Ravenous***
3. Fairly hungry
4. Slightly hungry
5. Neutral
6. Pleasantly satisfied
7. Full
8. ***Stuffed***
9. ***Bloated***
10. ***Nauseous***

Here's a simple exercise I teach in my live seminars that you may find useful to do for yourself:

Resetting the Thermostat

1. Stop for a moment and remember a time when you were really hungry, or even starving. What did it feel like? Where in your body did you feel it? Really remember it in every detail now.

2. Next, remember a time when you felt completely stuffed. What did that feel like? Where in your body did you feel it? Again, remind yourself exactly what that felt like now.

3. When you're ready, compare the difference between the two feelings. What's it like to feel really hungry? What's it like to feel stuffed? Keep going back and forth between the two extremes about ten times to help your body to remember and recalibrate.

It may not feel like much is happening when you first do this exercise, but your body and unconscious mind are beginning an important process of recalibrating your inner signals. Each time you repeat it, it becomes easier to notice when you are truly hungry and stop eating as soon as you are full.

Changing the Habits of a Lifetime

I was with a friend of mine recently who had been a serial dieter but only seemed to be getting a little bit fatter and a lot more frustrated each year.

In less than six months, he has lost fifty-six pounds using my system. At first he wasn't sure if it was working, but he stuck to it and after a couple of weeks he noticed his clothes felt looser. He hadn't even done any of the hypnosis techniques—I had simply taught him the four golden rules that I have just taught you and he started using them. When we were at dinner recently he only ate about half of his meal—a delicious-looking plate of pasta in a rich, creamy sauce. When I asked him if there was anything wrong with his food, he replied, "No—it's delicious. But ever since you taught me that damn system, I can't seem to overeat anymore."

He told me that he didn't even have to think about applying it—it had become second nature to him in a matter of weeks. This is typical of the progression most people experience. In the beginning, you need to consciously learn and apply each step. Then it begins to get easier and easier, and before you know it, you just do it because it's natural—the way your body was designed to eat.

When it comes to losing weight and keeping it off, habit is most people's worst enemy. For you, it will be different. We're going to recondition your habits and make them work for you. The hypnosis techniques throughout this book and on the CD will reinforce those new habits as the changes begin happening almost immediately.

Resigning from the "Clean Plate Club"

Why would anyone eat if they weren't hungry?

One of Professor Wansink's experiments involved drilling two holes in the bottom of a table at a university restaurant and placing two bowls with tubes attached over the holes. The plan was that researchers would be able to refill the bowls secretly without the diners noticing. On the opposite side of the table, he set two ordinary bowls.

When the students came into the cafeteria, he told them that he was conducting an experiment into the quality of the soup. In reality, the exact same soup was served to everyone. The difference was that the diners eating from the bowls with the holes in them didn't notice that as they ate the soup their bowls were being gradually refilled. Instead of listening to the signal from their stomach that said they had enough, they just kept on eating until they finished what was in the bowl. The result was that on average they ate a whopping 73 percent more than the other diners!

One of the main habits that gets in the way of listening to your body is being a lifetime member of what I call the "clean plate club." Members of this club think that unless they finish everything put in front of them, they are somehow misbehaving.

But eating everything on your plate whether you're still hungry and enjoying it or not is basically giving permission for your weight to be controlled by some kid who's being paid six dollars an hour at McDonald's. Let's face it: you wouldn't let a sales clerk tell you how much to spend on clothes, would you?

Like most kids, I was told by my parents to eat everything on my plate because "there are starving children in India." Don't underestimate the subtle power of this guilt trip, especially if it was instilled at a formative age. Eventually, of course, I realized that it was a con. I used to say, "How does me being overweight help the starving children? Shall I take a picture of myself fat and send it to them with a note saying, 'At least you know the food isn't going to waste'"?

Let me put this one to rest once and for all—contrary to popular parental opinion, eating everything on your plate has been shown to do nothing to contribute to the well-being of starving children in Africa, India, or China. If you really want to play your part in putting an end to world hunger, learn to manage your eating so that you eat when you're hungry, enjoy every mouthful, and stop when you think you're full. You'll wind up eating so much less that there'll be more for everyone else.

Of course, some members of the clean plate club aren't so concerned about world hunger—they feel guilty leaving a half-eaten chicken breast on their plate. But no matter how hard you try to resuscitate the other half of the chicken breast, it isn't coming back to life! Now, I don't know about you, but I find it difficult to imagine a chicken sitting up in chicken heaven looking down on you in judgment because you left part of his body on your plate.

Another popular excuse I hear from people is that it would be insulting to the chef if they left any food uneaten. For this one, I find the easiest thing is to blame me. Just tell them you used my hypnosis CD and that while you would love to eat the extra six portions of mashed potatoes in gravy, I have somehow messed with your mind and you can now only eat half as much as you used to! Of course it's important not to waste money, so sometimes you might want to take what you haven't eaten and keep it for later. However, remember *later* means only when you are truly hungry.

One of the simplest ways to give up your membership in the clean plate club for good is simply to deliberately leave a bit of food on your plate, even if it's just one little bit. In this way, you are sending a new message to your unconscious mind, letting it know for sure that you are changing. Once you've broken the spell (by leaving a little food on your plate each time you eat), you'll feel comfortable eating only until you feel full, even if it means leaving half or more of the food on your plate. You'll have less food in your stomach and more control in your life.

(And if you get hungry again later, don't worry—get another plate and leave some food on that one as well!)

The Magic Weight-Loss Elixir

There is one other thing that will support you in your efforts to eat only when you are hungry and stop as soon as you even suspect you are full. Our bodies are made up of roughly 75 percent water, and that increases to nearly 85 percent in the all-important area of brain tissue. When the inner mechanism in our body that regulates water levels senses any sort of current or impending shortage, your body goes into selective water rationing mode. The brain gets first call on the water supply, with each internal organ receiving just enough water to maintain basic functioning.

According to Dr. F. Batmanghelidj, author of the groundbreaking work *Your Body's Many Cries for Water*, many of the aches and pains that people experience on a daily basis, including hunger, are actually the preliminary effects of dehydration. This is one of the reasons why sometimes no matter what you eat, it doesn't feel as though it "hits the spot."

Because it's virtually impossible to tell the difference between this thirst signal and authentic hunger, it's a good idea to make your first response to hunger pangs a fresh glass of water. If you're not hungry afterward, it was thirst; if you still are, dig in!

What to Expect in the Next Two Weeks

1. It will feel a little weird

Some people tell me that at first they felt a little bit self-conscious eating slowly and consciously chewing each mouthful, as though other people were staring at them. As the saying goes, "You would worry less about what other people thought of you if you knew how seldom they did." Most people are so caught up in their own heads they don't even notice what's going into their mouths, let alone what's going on with yours.

Also, people who know you as a serial dieter may notice the pizza, bacon, or chocolate on your plate and smirk, thinking that you've "fallen off another diet."

This time, the last laugh will be on them. As it becomes easier and easier to eat consciously, your food will taste better and better and you will enjoy the wonderful feeling of satisfaction that comes from being in control of your eating.

In a society as filled with mixed messages about eating and body image as ours, what is considered "normal" may be a long way from what is actually natural. While it may feel a bit odd at first to reprogram your body to eat in a new, more intuitive way, it is important to recognize you are actually moving toward a more natural way of eating. This is why it is sustainable—unlike diets, which go against your natural urge to eat when you are hungry and stop when you are full, the simplest weight-loss system in the world works *with* your body.

2. You will feel good

One of the most consistent benefits people report from using the simplest weight-loss system in the world is that they feel better—better in their bodies and better in themselves.

Here's what to expect:

- For the first time in ages you will feel more in control around food.

- The pressure of worrying about what to eat and when will be gone. It will be liberating to know you are free from the slavery of obsessing about food.

- You will see that it truly is possible for you to lose weight easily.

- You will realize that slim people are not different from you. We are all the same in our ability to lose weight.

In fact you will be amazed at how easy it is!

Because you are not spending so much energy worrying about food you will have more energy available for your life. This extra energy is one of the signs that the system is working perfectly.

3. You will wonder how well it's working

People who have successfully used this system often say that within the first couple of weeks they weren't sure if it was working. Whether you feel like you are eating more than before, or that you're not eating nutritionally balanced meals, or even like nothing much is different . . .

Relax! As long as you are following the four golden rules, it's working.

It's normal to have doubts simply because you are doing something very different from what you have done before. Soon, as you begin to notice increased levels of energy, a slight change in how your clothes fit, and a general sense of well-being in your body, you will realize that everything is working perfectly. Remember, you have already tried all sorts of other systems, diets, or techniques and they haven't worked, or they've only worked for a short time. By committing to my system for the next two weeks, you've got nothing to lose except weight.

4. You will at some point forget to follow my instructions and break at least one if not all four of the golden rules

It's important for you to know that you *will* have a slip or two along the way, shoving in a sandwich on the run, gorging yourself on cookies, eating to calm your nerves, or even going on a full-out binge.

At this point you have a choice:

You can beat yourself up (as you've done in the past) and give up, telling yourself that you're a worthless piece of crap and you're never going to change.

Or:

You can *relax*, smile, remind yourself that I told you this would happen, and return to eating what you want when you are hungry, consciously enjoying each mouthful, and stopping when you think you are full. No matter what happens, always go back to following my instructions. Give this system a fair chance and you'll be glad of it for the rest of your life.

Weighing Yourself

Let me offer you one final note of caution. Over the years that I have been working with weight-loss clients, I have noticed how many people are absolutely obsessed with weighing themselves. Some do it every day; some even do it after every meal, treating the scales like the lottery, expecting to see that suddenly they have lost thirty pounds since lunchtime.

> *You cannot get an accurate reading of your weight loss by checking every day.*

Each time you climb on to those scales, all you are doing is setting yourself up to feel bad. Everybody's weight goes up and down all the time—even slim people. In fact, naturally thin people rarely if ever weigh themselves. Most of them couldn't tell you what they weigh if you paid them.

Because weight can fluctuate as much as ten pounds up or down from environmental factors, water retention, and even atmospheric pressure, it is actually the least reliable measure on the road to becoming thin. So it is important that you *do not weigh yourself* for the next two weeks.

I actually recommend that you give up the scales for life—you'll know you're thin because you look great and you feel wonderful. However, if you absolutely must weigh yourself, leave at least *two* weeks between each weighing.

When an airplane flies from one place to another, it doesn't fly in a straight line—it's always adjusting its course. Despite the fact that it's off course as much as 90 percent of the time, it always knows where it's going.

It's the same with losing weight—while some days will be better than others and sometimes you will feel more confident about your weight than others, if you keep your eye on the prize and keep following the guidelines, *you will lose weight* and keep it off, for as long as you use this system.

Can It Really Be This Simple?

Yes! Let's review the four elements of the system:

1. Eat when you're hungry.

2. Eat only what you want, never what you think you "should."

3. Eat consciously and enjoy every mouthful.

4. Stop when you think you're full.

That is all you have to do in order to lose weight and keep it off for life. And if you're truly ready to be thin, I can make it even simpler for you. If you change only one thing about the way that you eat, do this:

Consciously enjoy every mouthful.

By focusing on this one element of the system, everything else will fall into place, because:

- You can't and won't get the full enjoyment out of your food if you're not truly hungry.

- You can only truly enjoy your food when you choose only foods you truly enjoy.

- Your food will stop being enjoyable if you don't stop eating when your body is full.

FREQUENTLY ASKED QUESTIONS ABOUT

"The Simplest Weight-Loss System in the World"

Q. What if I can't tell when I am full?

In his book *Achieving Vibrance*, Gay Hendricks teaches about a mechanism in the body he calls "the V spot," which is located in your solar plexus, just below your rib cage and toward the center of your body. This is actually a muscle that is designed to control the flow of food to the stomach. Unfortunately, it's not a very strong muscle for most of us! However, as you become more and more sensitive to your body's signals, you can actually feel the V spot close off when your body has had enough food.

In the meantime, just stop if you suspect you might be full, knowing that it doesn't matter if you're wrong—you can always start eating again if it turns out your body is still hungry.

Q. It's a huge relief to eat when I'm hungry,
but I feel guilty eating whatever I want.
Can I do one without the other?

No, no, no, no, and no. One of the worst consequences of the diet conspiracy is that serial dieters are continually looking over their shoulders for the food police, lest they be caught enjoying food and sent back to starvation purgatory. Your body was made to run on food, and it will always tell you what it needs once you learn to listen.

Every time you eat something you don't really want, you're reinforcing the idea that someone other than you and your body knows best about what you need—and while that's great news for the advertising industry, it's a recipe for disaster when it comes to losing weight.

Q. I can't seem to quit the clean plate club
no matter how hard I try—do you have
any further suggestions?

It sounds as though you are still trying to "willpower" yourself thin, which is a bit like trying to hammer in nails with nothing but a screwdriver. It's not that it's not a useful tool, but rather that it's the wrong tool for the job at hand. By using your imagination instead of your will, you'll find it nearly effortless to leave food on your plate and out of your stomach.

If you're really stuck, try this: cut off a few bites of food before you start eating and either throw them away or sweep them onto a spare plate and ask your waiter or waitress to take it away. Then you can eat everything that's left on your plate (providing you're actually hungry).

If after all that you still find yourself feeling guilty about leaving that half-eaten chicken breast on your plate, you can use the tapping technique that I will share with you in chapter 6 to eliminate the unnecessary guilt and move on with your healthy body and healthier life!

Claire's Story

Claire Singh
Lost 112 pounds

Before

After

My weight had been a problem for most of my adult life. If you'd asked me what I ate in a day, I'd have told you, but I'd have unintentionally left things out because I ate without thinking. I didn't register it. I didn't think about whether I was hungry or not.

My mom paid for Paul's workshop as a Christmas present. I thought I'd go, as I had nothing to lose. I'll never forget that day. It was so simple and so inspiring, such a huge revelation, as if someone had just woken me up and said, "Here are the answers."

For the first time in my life, I started thinking about the food I ate, before and while eating it. At the same time, I started going to the gym, where I was helped by Mike, my personal trainer. The exercise seemed like a natural accompaniment to my new, "normal" lifestyle.

I now view food in a completely different way. I know that food is fuel for the body, not a life crutch. Ever since attending Paul's workshop, I've eaten a lot less. I think about what I eat and become full more easily. I don't eat junk food, and I've improved my cooking skills. Not only do I feel better from losing so much weight, but I'm also more in tune with my body, and no longer suffer from bad health generally and a poor digestive system.

I still listen to Paul's CD. It's useful for refocusing my mind, and it's supportive. I'll always be grateful for the life-changing experience. It's like someone said, "Here's the key to the rest of your life . . ."

Claire lost an average of 36 pounds over 12 months. Generally, people who use this program lost, on average, 1–2 pounds per week.

3.

Program Your Mind to Slim Your Body

The Habits of a Lifetime

I know there have been many times in the past when you've done your best to eat sensibly, but no matter how hard you tried, you couldn't stick with it. And you probably thought that in some way it was your fault—if only you had more willpower, you wouldn't be overweight.

Based on the latest scientific data, I can address that issue once and for all:

Rubbish!

The truth is that it's nearly impossible to break a habit with willpower alone—you have to reprogram your mind. With the right programs in place, doing the right thing is easy; with the wrong programs running your mind, it's virtually impossible.

Over the years, I have helped people change lifelong compulsions in a matter of minutes and proved that even the most die-hard addiction will succumb to effective reprogramming. Yet until you've experienced it for yourself, this may seem a bit different. After all, if lasting changes can happen this quickly and this easily, why haven't you been able to do it in the past?

It all boils down to a simple psychological rule:

Your imagination is far more powerful than your will.

To give yourself a quick experience of this, imagine a piece of chocolate cake (or your favorite food) in front of you. Next, tell yourself with all your willpower that you are not going to eat it. Then imagine the taste of that chocolaty icing as it melts on your tongue. Can you feel your will weakening yet?

Next, once again imagine that piece of chocolate cake (or your favorite food) in front of you. Now, imagine the cake is covered in maggots—slimy, wriggling maggots. Notice the foul smell emanating from the maggots (or is it the cake?). Has the cake lost some of its appeal?

That's the power of your imagination in action. In fact, it's through your imagination that you actually make all your best decisions about what you are going to eat. When you read the menu in a restaurant, you mentally taste all the food in your mind before you decide what to have. That's why restaurants go to such trouble to describe their food in appetizing terms. For example, which would you rather have for dinner this evening: "Medallions of swordfish lightly sautéed and served in a delicate lemon sauce" or "dead fish"?

The Focus Factor

Take a moment now to ask yourself:

What do I want in relation to my body?

If you're like most people, you answered something like "to lose weight" or "to get rid of my love handles" or "to not be so fat."

One of the most basic psychological rules in life is, "You always get more of what you focus on." Yet in each of the examples above, your mind has to focus on what you *don't* want in order to make sense of it—the weight you want to lose, the "love handles" that you secretly hate, or the fat you want to leave behind. This not only reinforces the image people have of themselves as fat, it tends to leave them feeling helpless, hopeless, and unmotivated.

When you redirect your focus exclusively onto what you want—a slim, fit, healthy body—you are sending a message to your unconscious mind to find and explore every possible opportunity to move toward your goal. By clarifying and vividly imagining exactly what it is you want for yourself, you are beginning the process of training your mind and body to give it to you. The more specific you are, the better this works. If you just say, "I'd like to be thinner," your mind might interpret that as meaning you want to lose one pound. So describe exactly what it is that you want.

For example:

I want to lose fifty pounds in the next four months.

Or:

I want to feel comfortable in a size eight dress.

Or my personal favorite:

I want to look great naked!

Self-Image and the Self-Fulfilling Prophecy

Remember, all you need to do to reach your goal is:

1. Eat when you're hungry.

2. Eat what you actually want.

3. Eat consciously and enjoy each mouthful.

4. Stop when you think you're full.

So why keep reading?

Because the techniques that follow will make the whole process happen even more easily and allow you to feel significantly better about yourself as well. In other words:

> *We are not only what we eat,*
> *but what we think as well.*

In the 1960s the famous plastic surgeon Maxwell Maltz found that after many of his operations, the self-esteem and confidence levels of his patients rose dramatically. However, for a few people the operations didn't seem to make any difference. After a great deal of exploration, Dr. Maltz concluded that those patients who didn't experience a change in their levels of well-being were "scarred on the inside." They saw themselves as unworthy, bad, or hopeless, and the fact that their appearance had changed on the outside made no difference to the image they held of themselves on the inside. They had what he called "an impoverished self-image."

Your self-image is how you see yourself in your imagination. It's the blueprint that determines everything about you, from how motivated, intelligent, and confident you are willing to let yourself be to how much weight you are willing to carry around with you or to lose.

The reason our self-image has such a powerful influence on our behavior is that it is self-reinforcing. For example, we've all met people who are not classically good-looking but have an aura of attractiveness. Because they think of themselves as attractive they carry themselves well, dress to bring out their most attractive features, and have the confidence to speak to anyone. This self-confidence makes them attractive to others, who respond positively to them, which reinforces their image of themselves as attractive.

Equally, there are plenty of people who think of themselves as unattractive, and unconsciously sabotage any attempts to appear attractive. After all, if you truly believe you are unattractive, why take the time to dress mutton up as lamb? However, if you don't do what it takes to represent yourself at your best, people will inevitably find you unattractive.

Either way, your self-image has worked perfectly, "proving" itself right by guiding you to act consistently with who you believe yourself to be.

Nearly every overweight person has a self-image that says they will always be fat. While they may say they would prefer to be thin, they often think that thin people are somehow different from them, and the goal seems almost unattainable.

How do you change the pattern?

By getting into the habit of focusing your attention on what you actually *do* want. Like it or not, you're going to have to get used to thinking of yourself with an attractive body!

See Yourself Slim

Recent scientific research in the United States and Europe has conclusively shown that visualization techniques dramatically enhance the ability to lose weight. As you vividly imagine yourself slim and rehearse your path to your ideal weight, you send a message to your brain that affects your energy levels, your motivation, and your metabolism. Those changes cause physical sensations, which in turn affect your thoughts and emotions, which in turn reinforce the programming you are giving your brain. It's a positive feedback system, and every element of the system gets to feel good as you lose weight.

As I guide you through these next two exercises, I am going to be instructing you to visualize. This is something everyone already has the ability to do. To prove this to yourself, answer the following questions:

1. What does your front door look like?

2. What color is it?

3. Which side is the handle on?

In order to answer any of these questions, you had to visualize—to go into your imagination and make pictures. Now, for 99 percent of people, these mental images will not be as real as reality—and that's a good thing. People who can't tell the difference between the pictures in their head and what they see in the world are in trouble.

Your Perfect Body

Here's a simple but powerful exercise that will train your unconscious mind to help you lose weight and keep it off. Before you do this exercise, read through all the steps first.

1. Stop for a moment and imagine you are watching a movie of a thin, happy, confident you.

2. Watch that thinner you doing the things that you do in your daily life and accomplishing them with ease. Imagine this new you eating just the right amount, moving their body regularly, and handling their emotional needs quickly and easily.

   - How does that other you talk to themself?
   - What kind of voice tone do they use?
   - How do they carry themself?
   - How do they move?

3. If the movie is not yet exactly how you want things to be, make the adjustments that make you feel great. Allow your intuition to be your guide.

4. When you are satisfied with the other you, step into it. Take the new perspective and behaviors into you.

5. Now run the movie and imagine being in all of your daily situations and view them from your new perspective. Think through what it's like to have this new perspective and what it will help you to achieve. How are things going to be so much better now?

Repetition, Repetition, Repetition

Remember, repetition is the key to success. When we repeat an action, a neural pathway is created in the brain and each repetition reinforces it. As you think of yourself as slim and healthy, you are sending signals to your unconscious mind to behave, to feel, and to eat like a slim person. As your body gets lighter you will feel more sensitive, more energetic, and more alive.

Do this exercise every morning and before long, it will become a healthy habit. The more you do this, the sooner you will start to feel better and change the way you feel about yourself for the better. Each time you do it, you will be one step closer to your ideal weight.

This exercise focuses your mind on your target, making it more powerful and more and more compelling, so that every time you say no to the foods you no longer wish to eat and yes to those foods you actually want, you will feel more of this delightful lightness and know you are one step closer to your ideal weight.

In addition, each time you listen to the special hypnosis CD, you will be reinforcing all the gains you make each time you take the time to see yourself slim.

FREQUENTLY ASKED QUESTIONS ABOUT

"Program Your Mind to Slim Your Body"

Q. What do I do if I'm having trouble seeing myself in my mind's eye?

Just keep listening to the CD and let me do the work. You wouldn't go to a restaurant and expect to cook your own dinner, would you? All you have to do is sit back, relax, and let the powerful suggestions on the hypnosis CD do their job. By the time you've listened at least once a day for at least two weeks, your mind and body will have already begun to change for the better.

Q. I find that I fall asleep listening to the CD. Will it still work for me?

Yes—in some ways it will work even more easily than when you stay awake and listen consciously!

Any new mother knows that no matter how deeply

she sleeps with one part of her mind, another part of her mind will wake her up immediately if her baby starts to cry.

Similarly, even while your body sleeps, your unconscious mind is listening. All the positive messages from the CD are going directly into your unconscious, reinforcing your new, healthy relationship with food each and every time you listen.

As an additional resource, I have created an online club at www.mckenna.com where you can get complete support in losing weight and keeping it off for life. As a member, you'll be able to watch mini-movies demonstrating each of the techniques featured in the book and receive coaching from me and others who have successfully lost weight and kept it off using this system. Please note, becoming a member is NOT necessary in order for you to succeed; however, many people have reported how much they appreciate being a part of a community of like-minded people as they move forward with their own weight-loss goals.

Christopher's Story

Christopher Wilde
Lost 211 pounds

Before   **After**

I knew things were bad when I realized that I was just waiting to die. I felt my body couldn't take any more punishment and it seemed just a matter of time before it gave up. I had just lost both my parents to cancer, I was struggling to find a good job after spending eighteen years in one I hated, and I was facing financial ruin. I barely had the energy to fight any more.

Just when I was giving up, I discovered Paul

McKenna's weight loss system *I Can Make You Thin*. I
didn't know it at the time, but that discovery saved
my life. I've done plenty of diets in the past and I
have lost large amounts of weight but it always came
back—plus a lot more. After twenty-five years of
struggling with my weight, it was suddenly easy with
this system to lose weight and keep it off.

I was 386 pounds when I started. I now weigh 175
pounds. I lost that weight in fourteen months. When I
look back I can hardly believe how much things have
changed. Not only did the system help me to lose all
that weight, but it helped me build the confidence to
face up to my problems and deal with them. I have
sorted out my financial problems and I've found
myself a great career—instead of driving buses and
trucks, I assess the qualifications of drivers, and I am
much happier in my work. And I've kept the weight
off!

Christopher lost 211 pounds over 14 months.
Generally, people who used this program lost, on
average, 1–2 pounds per week.

4.

Overcoming Emotional Eating

Recognizing Emotional Hunger

One of the most common mistakes people make when they first start out on my system is to confuse emotional hunger with physical hunger. This is because until we become more attuned to our bodies, the two feel remarkably similar.

In fact, the number-one reason people eat when they're not hungry is to cover up a negative emotion or to fill an emotional hole. That's why you can sometimes find yourself eating and eating without getting full—you were never hungry for food in the first place.

Perhaps you had an argument and had some chocolate to make yourself feel better, or you got home after a long, hard day and decided to cheer yourself up with some ice cream. Maybe you just were feeling bored and suddenly decided that a plate of cheese and crackers would hit the spot. But as my friend Michael Neill says, "There aren't enough cookies in the world to make you feel loved and whole."

Here are a couple of pointers to help you make a clear distinction every time:

1. Emotional hunger is sudden and urgent; physical hunger is gradual and patient

Have you ever had the experience of having a sudden, desperate craving for food?

If you track back in your mind, you'll find that only moments before the "hunger" arrived, you were having an argument with yourself in your mind. In order to not deal with whatever feelings are going on in the body, people learn to bury those feelings with food.

Physical hunger, on the other hand, is gradual. You may notice a gentle griping in your tummy, or even a deep rumbling. If you continue to ignore your hunger, you'll probably experience light-headedness or even sadness, anger, or tiredness. The earlier you learn to pick up on your body's hints that it needs fuel, the easier it will be to separate these two signals.

2. Emotional hunger cannot be satisfied with food; physical hunger can

If you are eating and eating and never feeling satisfied, it's because you don't need food—you need to change your feelings. When you're hungry for good feelings (or at least a temporary masking of bad feelings), no amount of food will do the trick. This is an additional way in which emotional hunger differs from physical hunger— when you address the root cause of emotional hunger, it doesn't come back again four hours later!

Regardless of its specific manifestations, the feelings that underlie emotional hunger invariably come down to just one thing:

Inescapable stress

According to the latest thinking among researchers into craving and addiction, "inescapable stress" is the ongoing sense that nothing can be done to reduce the amount of stress you are experiencing in your life. That seemingly inescapable stress may take the form of a bad marriage, a chronic illness, or stress at work. It can even be caused by guilt or shame—the regret for something that happened in the past that can never be undone.

In his excellent book *The Craving Brain*, Dr. Ronald Ruden points out that the experience of inescapable stress actually changes "the landscape of the brain," creating a physiological craving for substances (like food and/or alcohol) that will allow us to move our experience of stress into the background. In essence, food becomes a Band-Aid that provides temporary relief without actually leading to any improvement in the situation that caused the stress in the first place.

Based on this cutting-edge research, we now have a "magic pill" to help you lose weight:

Control your response to stress and you will no longer want or need to overeat.

As we have already learned, the mind and body are intimately linked. Recent scientific research has shown that our thoughts have a significant effect upon our health and well-being. We can change biological processes in the body through our imagination and we can certainly change our feelings and moods. As you reprogram your mind and develop your ability to respond to stress, you will actually change the neurochemical landscape of your brain.

In this next exercise, we are going to use a simple associational technique to create an inner sense of calm inside your body—the same sense of calm and peace you used to give yourself by overeating. By repeatedly doing this exercise and reenforcing it with the hypnotic suggestions on the CD, you will be able to lower your stress levels and gently eliminate your emotional hunger pangs without the worry, angst, or struggle most people experience.

The Calm Anchor

Before you do this exercise, read through all the steps first.

1. Remember a time when you felt really, really calm—at peace and in control. Fully return to it now, seeing what you saw, hearing what you heard, and feeling how good you felt. (If you can't remember such a time, imagine how wonderful it would feel to be totally at peace— if you had all the ease, comfort, and self-control you could ever need.)

2. As you keep running through this experience in your mind, make the colors brighter and richer, the sounds crisper, and the feelings stronger. When you are feeling these good feelings, squeeze the thumb and middle finger of your right hand together. You are associating this particular pressure in this particular place with this particular emotion. Run through this memory several times until you feel a lovely sense of inner peace and calm.

3. Now go through this relaxing memory at least five more times while continuing to squeeze your thumb and middle finger together to really lock in these good feelings. You will know you have done it enough when all you need to do is squeeze your fingers together and then

you can easily remember the feelings of calm and relaxation spreading through your body.

4. Next, think about a situation that in the past you would have found mildly stressful. Once again, squeeze your thumb and middle finger together. Feel that calm feeling spreading through your body and imagine taking it with you into that stressful situation. Imagine everything going perfectly, exactly the way you want. See what you'll see, hear what you hear, and feel how good it feels to be so much calmer and in control in this situation.

5. Now, still squeezing your thumb and finger together, remember that calm feeling of being in control and once again imagine being in that situation that used to seem stressful. This time, imagine a few challenges occurring and notice yourself handling all the challenges perfectly. See what you'll see, hear what you hear, and feel how good it feels to be so much calmer and in control in this situation.

6. Stop and think about that situation now. Notice the difference from only a few minutes ago. Do you feel less stressed and more in control? If not, just repeat the exercise until you do!

Each time you do this exercise, it will become easier and easier to experience feelings of relaxation and calm "at your fingertips."

Your Harshest Critic

One of the most common sources of inescapable stress is a secret many people carry with them throughout their lives:

> ***Self-loathing—feeling helpless, hopeless, worthless, and unloved***

I am continually amazed at the self-abuse that most people put themselves through at the start of each day. They'll look at themselves in the mirror in the morning, say, "fat face, fat arms, fat thighs, fat butt," and then go through their day wondering why they don't feel good about themselves.

In my weight-loss seminars I do an exercise where I help people stop the self-abuse and start to appreciate themselves. I ask for a volunteer to look into a mirror and share their internal criticism out loud with the group. Once, I was doing this exercise with a lovely looking lady who saw herself in the mirror and immediately blurted out, "Big fat pig."

Of course everyone burst out laughing because they could so easily identify with her. When I asked her what she would do if someone walked up to her in the street and said that to her, she replied that she would probably hit them. She wouldn't take it from someone else, but she'd readily insult herself every time she looked in the mirror.

Possibly the most famous guideline for effective living in Western civilization is the so-called golden rule, which is generally expressed in some version of "Do unto others as you would have done unto you." My candidate for a "platinum rule" is this:

Do unto yourself as you would have others do unto you.

If anyone else insulted us as openly and crudely as we insult ourselves ("I'm such a stupid idiot," "I'm so useless," "I'm such a waste of space," "God, I'm pathetic," etc.) or punished us as unforgivingly as we punish ourselves ("I can't believe I ate dessert—that's it! I'm going to work out until I throw up!"), we would be up in arms, protesting at the injustice and inhumanity of such cruel and unusual treatment.

But when we treat ourselves that way, we put up with it—mostly because nobody ever told us we didn't have to. Until you realize that there are healthy alternatives to motivating yourself to lose weight by beating yourself up for being fat, you will find it virtually impossible to measure up to your own unrealistically high standards. Fortunately, by seeing self-loathing for what it is, you lessen its power over you and make it possible to address it directly instead of attempting to stuff it down with food.

As you begin to see yourself as capable, lovable, and intrinsically worthy, you will continue to feel the pangs of emotional hunger. When you are feeling low, it is commonplace that friends and family can see your strengths and value even when you do not. We can use this fact to begin the process of loving and valuing ourselves. Here's an exercise to help you begin to change the patterns of self-loathing that most of us have been carrying throughout our lives.

Somebody Who Loves You

Before you do this exercise, read through all the steps first.

1. Close your eyes and think of someone who loves or deeply appreciates you. Remember how they look, and imagine they are standing in front of you now.

2. Gently step out of your body and into the body of the person who loves you. See through their eyes, hear through their ears, and feel the love and good feelings they have as you look at yourself. Really notice in detail what it is that they love and appreciate about you. Recognize and acknowledge those amazing qualities that perhaps you hadn't appreciated about yourself until now.

3. Step back into your own body and take a few moments to enjoy those good feelings of knowing that you are loved and appreciated exactly as you are.

You can keep that inner feeling with you for hours and hours and rerun this exercise whenever you want to boost that feeling. The more you do it, the easier it becomes, and eventually it becomes almost automatic to love and feel loved.

The Natural Design of Your Body

Did you know that less than 1 percent of the women in the world even have the genetic potential for what is considered a "model figure"? Yet when I meet people who consider themselves to be overweight, they spend an inordinate amount of time comparing themselves to airbrushed magazine images of smiling, anorexically thin women and make themselves feel so bad they need to eat something in order to feel better!

Our bodies contain a natural blueprint for optimal health. Human beings are designed to be around five or six feet tall, and that's why we stop growing in our late teens. No one continues growing to twenty feet—it wouldn't be natural and it wouldn't be healthy. In the same way, we have a natural shape. If we get too much bigger or smaller than that, it's because we have interfered with the natural design of the body.

It is very common for people to tell me that they don't like their bodies and will do whatever they can to try to ignore them. What they don't realize is that it is important to pay attention: if you want to change how you look, you must first make peace with your natural body. In fact, the more you learn to accept your body as it is, the more you'll be amazed at how effortlessly it changes.

Here's the bottom line:

You've got to make friends with the body you have in order to get the body you want.

Of course you may be looking forward to thinner thighs or a flatter tummy, but it is this same body you are already in that is going to be fitter and slimmer, so you may as well begin making peace with it now.

Anorexia, Bulimia, and Body Dysmorphia

All of the techniques in this book can make a real difference in the way you feel about yourself and the actions you take. In fact many people with eating disorders have told me that the discipline of following this system and practicing the self-esteem exercises have really helped them. However, if you suspect or have been told that you are suffering from an eating disorder, you should *seek help from a qualified professional*.

Even though anorexics and bulimics are often painfully thin, they tell themselves how overweight they are and say all kinds of abusive things to themselves when they look in the mirror.

Some of them are able to telescope their vision onto some tiny aspect of themselves, focusing all their self-hate onto that one body part. Others are able to completely hallucinate, as if looking in one of those fun-house mirrors at the carnival that make you appear much taller or wider than you really are. This distorted self-image, commonly referred to as "body dysmorphia," keeps people from truly enjoying life or eating enough. At best it has dire health consequences; at worst it can be fatal.

I worked with a lovely-looking lady on TV who couldn't look at herself in the mirror without bursting into tears. She'd tried every kind of therapy and none of it had worked. Using the techniques that I am about to teach you, she overcame this horrible lifelong disorder. In less than an hour, she was able to look confidently at herself in the mirror and see herself as beautiful.

During the change process I asked her to remember a time when she had been paid a compliment. Try as she might, she couldn't think of a single one.

Her partner was present and I suggested she think of a time when he'd said something nice to her. "That'll be the day!" she said. He looked a little hurt and surprised and replied, "I say nice things to you all the time."

Before she had a chance to argue, I jumped in and said, "I believe him!"

Our self-image acts as a filter for what fits with who we think we are. Because she had such a poor self-image, whenever anybody said anything nice to her, she immediately dismissed it because it didn't fit with who she thought she was.

The sweetest moment in this session came at the end. Although she had been with her partner for several years and they had a child together, they had never married because she couldn't bear the thought of "all those people looking at me on my wedding day while I was so hideous."

After we had taken away the self-hate and she filled herself up with love, I asked her how she felt about getting married now. She turned, smiled at her partner, and said, "Well, someone will have to ask me." She was finally able to let in all the love that he had been trying to give her for years.

The Friendly Mirror

Everyone receives compliments and praise from time to time. Sometimes they may seem trivial, like "Hey, you're looking great" or "You look sharp today." At other times they may seem quite significant, like "You are so sexy," or "Do you know how much people respect you?"

Sincere, positive perceptions from others, which you may not have been able to see or fully appreciate from the point of view you had at the time, can be valuable in learning to appreciate your own qualities more fully and enhance your self-esteem now.

The next three techniques will help you to eliminate emotional hunger by enabling you to feel better and better about yourself every time you look in the mirror. Read through each technique several times until you know the steps, and then go and do it. The entire process will take no more than ten minutes, and can be repeated as often as you choose.

The Friendly Mirror—Part One

Before you do this exercise, read through all the steps first.

1. Think of somebody who you think likes what they see when they look at themselves. You don't have to know this for a fact, but you suspect that when they look in the mirror they say nice things about themselves.

2. Imagine your model of beauty is standing in front of you. Imagine how they look, their posture, and as much as you can about them.

3. Next, close your eyes and imagine stepping into them—right into their body. Copy their body posture exactly and see through their eyes, hear through their ears, and feel the confident, happy feelings of self-appreciation they have.

4. Take those good feelings and move them up to the top of your head and down to the tip of your toes, until you are totally covered in that good feeling.

5. Now, staying in touch with that good feeling, open your eyes and stare into your eyes. *Do not look at your body*—just keep staring into your eyes for at least two minutes. This exercise recalibrates the perceptual filter of your consciousness and allows your mind to see more clearly in the future.

When you get comfortable with Part One, you can move on to:

The Friendly Mirror—Part Two

Before you do this exercise, read through all the steps first.

1. Standing in front of a mirror with your eyes closed, recall a specific time when you were paid a compliment by someone you respect or trust. You don't necessarily have to have believed the compliment at the time but you do have to trust the sincerity of the person who said it. Run through the experience all over again.

2. As you recall the compliment, and the sincerity of the person who said it, pay particular attention to your feelings of trust and regard for the other person.

3. When you feel that as strongly as possible, open your eyes, look in the mirror, and really see what they saw. Allow yourself to see what someone else has seen and notice how that feels.

4. Finally, imagine taking a picture of yourself just like that. Imagine taking that picture right into your heart. Keep it there so that you can look at it whenever you want to remind yourself how good you can feel.

When you get comfortable with Part Two, you can move on to:

The Friendly Mirror—Part Three

Before you do this exercise, read through all the steps first.

1. Each day, spend at least one minute looking at your body in the mirror. In an ideal world, you will do this without clothes, but if that doesn't feel right at first, you may wear anything that reveals your basic shape.

2. Notice what thoughts come up, from "This is stupid" to "God, I hate my thighs" to "Hmmm . . . not bad—not bad at all!"

3. Send love, approval, and positive energy to the person in the mirror. Let them know that you're on their side, and that your love for them is not dependent on the size of their thighs.

Remember to use these techniques every day and don't be too surprised at how quickly you begin to notice the changes. For many people, just moving from self-hate to a state of neutral self-acceptance is life-changing. Eventually, you will get all the way to love, and then the changes become even more dramatic.

As you begin actively to meet your own emotional needs, you will find your emotional hunger begins to diminish. As it does, eating only when you are truly hungry for food will become easier and more natural. You will become noticeably more confident and charismatic. Day by day, you'll find yourself naturally doing things that you used to only dream of.

FREQUENTLY ASKED QUESTIONS ABOUT
"Overcoming Emotional Eating"

Q. I'm hungry all the time, and I've been told it's just something I'd have to get used to. Could it also be partly emotional?

I would go so far as to say it's completely emotional. Being overweight is nearly always a symptom, and inescapable stress is nearly always the cause.

Yet book after book and program after program attempt to address the issue by telling you what you should or shouldn't eat. That's like trying to fix a broken leg by telling the person they shouldn't have fallen down! Instead of going outside yourself and asking the so-called diet experts, "What should I eat?" you need to go inside and ask yourself, "What's eating me?"

The next time you're feeling overwhelmed, sad, angry, lonely, or scared, put on the CD or use the exercises in this chapter to create a sense of instant calm and give yourself some unconditional love and approval. If you still want to eat after that, it's probably because you're actually hungry!

Q. I feel like I'm making real progress with this,
but from time to time I feel overcome by a real
need to eat an entire box of cookies. What do
I do when I want to binge?

As some of your old patterns of overeating dissipate, it
is not unusual for the odd craving to arise. When it
does, you can proceed directly to chapter 6 and use the
techniques to eliminate the cravings immediately!

Maureen's Story

Maureen Edwards
Lost 280 pounds

Before   After

I was at a barbecue one day. It was packed with
people. I piled up my plate, then sat down in a chair
my sister pointed out for me. (I found out later she'd
got the biggest chair she could find, especially for
me. A white plastic chair.) Anyway, when I went to
get up again, I couldn't. I was wedged in, and it was
buckling underneath me. Everyone was laughing,
and I tried to laugh too, but I was humiliated. My
husband and another friend had to help me get

out, shattering the arms of the chair—buried in my 72-inch thighs!—in the process.

Sobbing in the car on the way home, I decided to do something. A friend had recommended the Paul McKenna CDs. I was prepared to try anything, though I secretly thought that, like everything else I'd tried, it probably wouldn't work. A little ray of hope kept me going.

The next day I got the CDs, went upstairs to play them, and I can honestly say that that's the day my life changed.

Now I take him to bed every night! I'm the manager of a gym these days, and take regular aerobics classes myself. Sometimes I think back to not even being able to reach around to wipe my own backside. I know that's disgusting but that's how big I was. I've gone from almost 420 pounds to under 140 pounds in two years. Every day I still feel great about how different life is. I help other people too. I'm the Mo in Motivation! If I can do it, anybody can.

Maureen lost 280 pounds over 24 months. Generally, people who used this program lost, on average, 1–2 pounds per week.

5

Make Exercise Easy and Supercharge Your Metabolism

Exploding the Myth of Metabolism

Have you ever heard someone say they can't lose weight because they have a "slow" metabolism?

Your metabolism is the speed at which your body produces energy. The faster your metabolism, the faster your body does everything, from adjusting your body temperature to growing your fingernails. And more important for our purposes, the faster it will burn off any excess fat, regardless of whether that fat comes from a hearty roast beef platter or your hips, thighs, and stomach.

The rate at which your metabolism is currently running is called your "basal metabolic rate," and it is the primary determinant of how many calories your body will burn off throughout the day.

One of the great myths of the weight-loss world is the myth of metabolism, which says: *Certain people will find it more difficult to lose weight than others because of their genetically predetermined basal metabolic rate.*

However, the latest scientific research shows that your metabolic rate is not fixed—it can and will change throughout your life in response to how you eat and use your body.

Dr. Susan Jebb is one of Britain's leading experts in the study of obesity. When discussing metabolism on one of my TV shows, she explained it like this:

"When people go on a diet, their metabolism does change. Your body recognizes it's not getting as much food, as much fuel as it needs. The reduction in metabolic rate you see when people are dieting is essentially a very sensible evolutionary response to times of famine. If food was scarce, it made good sense to conserve energy and so your metabolic rate decreases."

In other words, someone may really have a slow metabolism—but the reason it's so slow is because they've *slowed* it through endless dieting! In its effort to conserve energy when you're dieting, your body will slow all your energy systems down to a minimum. You'll feel sluggish and completely uninterested in exercise or any other physical activity.

To make matters worse, whatever lean muscle mass you do have will be consumed as your body literally eats itself to generate the extra energy it needs to function. So even if you are temporarily losing weight on the scale, you're not losing the right kind of weight—you're losing muscle.

Why is losing muscle bad? Because that lean muscle controls your basal metabolic rate—the number of calories your body can burn up for you while you're sitting in the office or home in bed.

There are very few "sure things" in life, but I want to offer you one here:

If you continue to diet, you will gain weight and keep it on for life.

On the flip side, when you eat whenever you are hungry, your body learns it has plenty of fuel. It cranks up your metabolism so that energy can be used quickly and efficiently. Because it knows the energy will be replenished as needed, it doesn't bother to store any additional fat reserves, and you not only look thin but are filled with energy as well.

In the rest of this chapter, I will show you not only how to speed up your metabolism but how to "supercharge" it too, enabling you to burn more fat and calories throughout the day and even while you sleep!

The Truth about Exercise

When I asked Dr. Jebb if there was a secret to supercharging your metabolism, she told me:

"All you have to do is stop starving yourself and move your body more and your metabolism will increase. And the very best way to boost your metabolism is to become more active. Simply sitting in a chair uses up more energy than lying down. Standing up uses more energy than sitting down. Walking or climbing stairs all increase your metabolism and your energy needs. You can almost double your basic metabolic rate by being very physically active and burning off a lot of extra energy."

In other words, regular exercise will nearly double the speed of your metabolism. But before you throw your hands up in horror, realize that "exercise" is simply this:

Anything you do that causes you to breathe more deeply than you normally would and/or causes your heart rate to speed up.

Can you think of any enjoyable ways to get your heart pumping and breathe more deeply than you are breathing now?

If so, you are already on your way to making exercise an easy and enjoyable part of your life.

When I ask people about exercise, they think about running on a track or pumping iron. It always makes me laugh when people tell me that they never exercise. "Don't you get out of bed in the morning?" I ask them. "How about walking around your home? Do you ever leave your apartment or house? Does somebody carry you or do you do it on your own two feet?"

The fact is, you already "exercise" all day every day, simply by moving your body. The key to supercharging your metabolism (and in so doing, speeding up the rate at which your body burns through calories and fat) is simply to move more than you are currently doing. While the biggest exercise myth in the world is the idea of "no pain, no gain," the reality of exercise is this:

No effort, no gain;
a little bit of effort, tremendous gain.

Now let's take a look at some of the additional benefits of exercise. Studies have shown that regular exercisers not only lose weight, but they feel great. This is because exercise releases one of the best stress-reducing drugs available—your own natural endorphins. Here's how it works.

Your body does not distinguish between an emotional threat and a physical one. So even when you're just worrying about bad things happening, your body prepares to protect itself by fighting or running away—but often there is no one to fight and nowhere to run to. The body gets worked up but cannot find a way to release its tension.

Each time you exercise, you are helping your body release the tension of the stress response, making it feel calmer, safer, and healthier. In addition, regular exercise triggers the body's natural impulse to rest, relaxation, and recuperation, also known as the *parasympathetic response*.

The parasympathetic response is the sweet, soft feeling you get in your muscles when you have finished some heavy work or vigorous movement.

You also feel a natural high caused by the release of endorphins, the body's natural opiates. That in turn positively affects your mood, making you emotionally clearer and more able to function well—to concentrate, to relax, and to sleep soundly.

So any time you're feeling less than your best, you can give yourself an easy, positive boost by simply taking ten to fifteen minutes of brisk exercise—any movement (including walking) that speeds up your heart rate and gets you breathing more deeply than you are breathing right now.

How to Fail

Getting exercise helps you to build muscle, lose fat, and feel great. It contributes to clearer skin, enhanced mental clarity, better athletic performance, and an increased sex drive. Certain hormones released during exercise have been shown to slow and even reverse the aging process.

So why aren't you already doing more of it?

Well, it's probably because in the past you thought about exercise and imagined yourself huffing and puffing on an exercise machine, listening to a maniacal aerobics instructor shouting "feel the burn," or looking into a wall-size mirror surrounded by people who look so much better than you that you just want to go home and throw up.

Or maybe you bought an exercise machine for yourself that was advertised on TV, and you began to feel better the moment you ordered it. A few days later it arrived and you eagerly unpacked it, sure that the body of the model from the ad would be yours in just a few weeks' time. But within a month or so, your New Year's or birthday resolution became the world's most expensive clothes rack. In fact, most people put more and more clothes onto their exercise machines until they're so completely hidden that they don't have to look at them anymore and remind themselves of what they're not doing.

In both cases the problem is that you have not yet linked pleasure to the thought of exercise.

It really is that simple—if you want to exercise regularly, you must enjoy moving your body, both as you're doing it and after. Until you deliberately root out your negative associations with exercise and install new positive ones, you will continue to tell yourself you "should" do it and beat yourself up for not listening.

As I guide you through this next exercise, we are going to make the idea of moving your body much more appealing, using the psychological power of vivid visualization and simple association to create a super-state of motivation to exercise that you can trigger whenever you want.

You are going to do this by creating a trigger, or anchor, that will put you in touch with feeling great whenever you want. Since you already created a "calm" anchor using the thumb and middle finger of your right hand, you may want to put this one on your left or even use a different finger if you like. It's easy and inconspicuous and you can do it anywhere.

Motivation Power—Part One

In a moment we are going to remember some times when you felt totally motivated, or anything else that you *really* enjoy doing. Then we are going to create an association between those feelings and this squeeze of your fingers by repeating them together, over and over again.

Before you do this exercise, read through all the steps first.

1. Rate on a scale of 1 to 10 how strong your motivation to exercise is: 1 is the weakest, 10 the strongest.

2. Think of something you are already motivated to do. It may be something you feel particularly passionate about, like your favorite hobby or pastime, a political cause, being with a loved one, or spending time with your family. If nothing springs to mind immediately, ask yourself, if you had won a lottery jackpot, how motivated would you be to go and collect the check? Or how motivated would you be to

save the life of your closest friend? Or if the most attractive person in the world asked you out on a date, how motivated would you be to say yes?

3. Whatever motivates you most right now, I'd like you to visualize the scene—seeing it through your own eyes as though it's here now. See again what you would see, hear what you would hear, and feel exactly how being motivated feels. Now notice all the details of the scene. Make the colors richer, bolder, and brighter. Make the sounds clearer and the feelings stronger. As the feelings build to a peak, squeeze together your finger and thumb.

4. Keep going through that motivational movie. As soon as it finishes, start it again, all the time feeling that motivation and squeezing your thumb and finger together. See what you saw, hear what you heard, and feel that motivation.

5. STOP! Relax your fingers. Move around a bit.

Are you ready to test your motivation trigger? Squeeze your thumb and finger together and relive that good feeling now. It's important to realize it may not feel as intense, but you can increase your feelings of motivation every time you do this exercise.

Motivation Power—Part Two

Before you do this exercise, read through all the steps first.

1. It's time to make the association between feeling motivated and moving your body. Squeeze your thumb and finger together and remember what it's like to feel motivated. Now imagine yourself moving your body easily and effortlessly throughout the day. Imagine things going perfectly, going exactly the way you want them to go, finding more and more opportunities to enjoy moving your body in enjoyable ways. See what you'll see, hear what you'll hear, and feel how good it feels. As soon as you have done that, go through it again, still squeezing together your finger and thumb, permanently associating motivation to exercise.

2. Finally, on a scale of 1 to 10, how motivated do you feel to move your body? The higher the number, the easier you will find it to incorporate exercise into your daily routine. The lower the number, the more you need to practice the preceding technique. You can also listen to the hypnosis CD that comes with this book as often as you like. The more you listen, the more motivated to exercise you will become.

Simple Steps to Success

Our bodies are made with muscles that are designed to be used. Because lots of us work at desks and travel by car, bus, and train, we don't use our muscles as much as our ancestors used theirs. We have inherited all the healthy genes for fitness and a fast-burning metabolism, but we've fallen out of the habit of using them as much or as often as we could.

In an interesting study, researcher and author Dr. James Hill discovered that the average number of steps taken per day by women between the ages of eighteen and fifty was only a little over 5,000. (For men, the average was closer to 6,000 steps a day.) Even more intriguingly, the study revealed that people who were overweight took 1,500 to 2,000 fewer steps a day than those who maintained a healthy weight.

Think about that for a moment—*only 2,000 extra steps a day can make the difference between being overweight and being slim!* That's about the distance it would take for you to walk four city blocks. The more steps you take, the more calories you use up, and the increased speed of your metabolism from those extra steps will continue to burn away your fat while you rest or sleep.

While some doctors recommend you maintain at least 10,000 steps a day, I have known people to make remarkable strides with their weight loss by increasing their step count to as much as 20,000 a day.

If you'd like to figure out how many steps you already walk each day, you can purchase a simple pedometer (step counter) at almost any sports store for a couple dollars. Just attach it to your clothing when you get started in the morning and find out how many steps you currently take in a typical day. Aim to increase the number of steps by 2,000 a week until you hit a comfortably maintainable target.

It's important to remember that no matter how much you want to change, it will still only happen one day at a time. You don't have to start a formal exercise program (unless you want to clear up your skin, be less moody, and have better sex), but you do have to move your body. Do it whenever you get the chance. Take the stairs instead of the elevator. Park farther away from the office and walk 2,000 extra steps to work. Move. Dance. Play sports. Have fun. You only have one body, so you might as well enjoy it!

FREQUENTLY ASKED QUESTIONS ABOUT

"Make Exercise Easy and Supercharge Your Metabolism"

Q. Can I lose weight without any exercise?

Absolutely. As long as you are eating when you're hungry, eating what you actually want, enjoying each mouthful, and stopping when you're full, you will lose weight.

But remember, it's virtually impossible not to exercise unless you're completely bedridden. (And even then you're probably breathing . . .) So given how easy it is to accelerate your weight loss by moving just a little bit more than you already do, why would you want to lose weight the slower way?

Q. How long will it take me to speed up my metabolism?

Your metabolism will begin to speed up the minute you begin following the four golden rules. By gently introducing exercise into your routine, it will speed up even more. But take it easy on yourself! I have noticed that when some people reach the desperation point where they decide they "have to lose weight immediately," they begin starving themselves, power walking, and going to the gym all on the same day. When these people don't lose weight immediately (because they are driving their body into survival mode), they decide that it's all too much and give up on the whole project.

Any task can be achieved if it's broken down into small enough chunks. That's why it's a good idea to choose a type and amount of exercise that you can succeed at easily and then increase it bit by bit each week. That way, you get to feel in control every step of the way.

Once you've succeeded the first three times, you'll continue doing it for life!

Yvonne's Story

Yvonne Meaney
Lost 91 pounds

Before   **After**

I had dieted often over the years. I'd lose weight, then put it all back on, plus extra. I got heavier and heavier; by 2005 I was over 225 pounds, unhappy and convinced I'd be fat for life.

My husband lost weight using Paul's book and CD, and nagged me to try it. I didn't think it would work for me. Then over Christmas I was sitting on the sofa with the cat on my lap, and I asked John to put on a DVD as there was nothing interesting on

TV. Sneakily, he put in Paul's Weight-Loss DVD and said, "Watch that!" I didn't want to disturb the cat so I gave in and watched. At least it would stop the nagging!

To my surprise the advice made sense, and I started following the four golden rules. When I began to lose weight I realized there was something to this system, so I read Paul's book.

The section on exercise encouraged me to start walking. I started with 2,000 extra steps a day and found I enjoyed it. I got quicker and went farther and ended up running. It seemed the more I did the lighter I became and the easier it got, so I did more . . . and had fun doing it.

Ten months later I had lost 91 pounds and I haven't looked back. Running is now part of my life and I've taken part in numerous races. Recently I completed my first full marathon and I'm planning to do more.

Using this system has been life-changing. It was never a struggle, I never binged or felt miserable. It has given me complete freedom around food. I've gone from "Couch Potato" to "Marathon Runner" and I'm happy the weight has gone for good!

Yvonne lost 91 pounds over 10 months. Generally, people who used this program lost, on average, 1–2 pounds per week.

6.

Craving Busters

How to Take Control of Your Cravings

One of the main concerns that people have about using my system is that I am going to somehow trick them into hating their favorite foods and they'll constantly feel that they are missing out. Nothing could be further from the truth—as you've already learned, in my system there are *no* forbidden foods. As long as you're hungry and you like it, it's yours.

However, if you can't stop once you start or you can't resist a food even when you're not hungry, then in that moment you are out of control. If you have to demolish the whole bar of chocolate or scarf down the entire bag of chips, the food is in charge and not you. The techniques in this chapter will help put you back in charge of your body, your eating, and your life.

Now, if you have ever had a craving, you know that it feels like it needs to be satisfied immediately. In addition, most cravings are for a specific food, like chocolate, pizza, or cheesecake, as opposed to a more general hunger.

Here's all you need to know:

Any craving you may have felt is a learned behavior.

That means you weren't born with it, and if you learned it, you can unlearn it, often in a matter of minutes.

There are two techniques in this chapter. If you are in the midst of a food craving, I'm about to share with you a startlingly simple way you can reduce or even eliminate that craving in less than two minutes. If you would like to reprogram your mind to stop a particular craving forever, you can skip ahead to the second technique.

The Tapping Technique

This amazing technique was developed by Dr. Roger Callahan, author of *Tapping the Healer Within.*

In one of the television programs I did on weight loss, we featured a lady named Lizzie who drank four liters of cola every single day. We asked her to take part in a dramatic experiment—to go "cold turkey" and stop drinking cola completely. The results were distressing. Lizzie experienced constant cravings, and after only a few days she had become depressed and extremely emotional.

At that point I called her and guided her through the tapping technique I am about to share with you. Amazingly, within a few minutes the crying and the cravings had completely stopped. For the first time she could remember, Lizzie felt in control. When the cravings came back, as I had told her might happen, she was now able to switch them off at will.

The first day she had to tap them away almost a dozen times. By the next day it was down to eight, and by the end of the week the cravings were coming up only one or two times a day. At the time of writing, Lizzie has not drunk cola once since she learned the tapping sequence you are about to learn. Better still, she hasn't even experienced a craving for more than two years.

If you are feeling a strong craving for a particular food right now and you want to reduce or even eliminate it immediately, just follow my instructions completely and your craving will vanish. This process may seem a bit strange at first, but it works. You will have to be able to really concentrate for a few minutes, as it is important that you continue thinking about the food you have chosen as you go through this process and reduce the craving.

What we are about to do involves tapping on certain acupuncture points on your body. The code for any craving is stored like a computer program in your brain. By thinking about the food you are craving while tapping on each point in exactly the sequence I am about to describe, you reset your brain's operating software to bypass your cravings so you can easily get on with your life.

Craving Buster—Number One

Tapping into the Thin Within

Before you do this technique, read through each step so that you know exactly what to do.

1. I want you get the biggest desire for your favorite craving food. Now, rate your craving on a scale of 1 to 10, with 1 being the lowest and 10 the highest. This is important, because in a moment we will find out how much you've reduced it. On a scale of 1 to 10, how strong is your craving?

2. Now take two fingers of either hand and tap about ten times under your collarbone while you continue to think about your craving.

3. Now tap under your eye ten times.

4. Now tap under your collarbone again.

5. Place your other hand in front of you and tap on the back of it between your ring finger and

your little finger. Continue to think about your craving food as you do this and each of the steps that follow:

- Close your eyes and open them.

- Keep your head still, keep tapping and look down to the right and then down to the left.

- Keep tapping and rotate your eyes round 360 degrees clockwise, and now 360 degrees counterclockwise.

Remember to keep thinking about the food you were craving as you do this!

- Now hum the first few lines of "Happy Birthday" out loud.

- Count out loud from 1 to 5.

- Once again hum the first few lines of "Happy Birthday" out loud.

6. Stop and check—on a scale from 1 to 10, what number is your craving at now?

If the craving hasn't completely gone yet, just repeat this sequence again until it does. It may take as many as two or even three times before you have completely eliminated the craving, although most people report getting their craving down to a manageable level on their first or second try. You may even find that it is gone completely.

If it ever comes back, you can repeat this process as often as you like, or go through Craving Buster Number Two to reprogram your craving away forever.

Craving Buster—Number Two

The Compulsion Destroyer

While the tapping technique you have just learned can be used to reduce and ultimately even eliminate cravings over time, this next technique can eliminate food compulsions forever in just a few applications. In fact, I regularly demonstrate this technique on television and in my seminars to help people who consider themselves to be chocolate "addicts" to become unwilling to eat chocolate ever again—in less than two minutes!

I am now going to show you how to do the same thing for yourself—how you can stop yourself from ever wanting to eat a particular food again. Most people choose chocolate, bread, cookies, or some other "treat" food that has turned from an occasional treat to uplift the spirits to a heavy anchor around your hips and thighs.

Remember, only do this next technique if you genuinely want to stop eating a particular food for good! If you just want to reduce your craving, go back to "Tapping into the Thin Within." Read through this technique in its entirety before you do it.

1. Think of a food you hate—one that really disgusts you. (A woman in one of my seminars who swore that she loved to eat everything finally agreed that she found the idea of eating a plate of human hair repulsive.)

2. Next, I want you to vividly imagine there is a big plate of the food you hate in front of you. Now imagine smelling and then eating the food that you hate, as you squeeze the thumb and little finger of either hand together. Really imagine the texture of it in your mouth as you squeeze your thumb and little finger together. Imagine the taste of it, squeezing your thumb and little finger together until you feel utterly revolted. When you are feeling a bit nauseated, stop and relax your fingers.

3. Next, I want you to think of the food that you are going to stop eating. When you think of it, notice that you can imagine what a plate of it looks like.

4. Now, make that picture of the food you like bigger, bigger and brighter. Make it huge, until it's bigger than you are, and make it even bigger than that. Continue making it bigger and bigger and bring it closer and closer and then pass it through you and out the other side. (Most people say that it feels a bit weird to pass the picture through your body—like when a ghost passes through someone's body in the Harry Potter stories.)

5. Ready? Squeeze your thumb and finger together and remember the taste of the food you hate, while at the same time imagining eating some of the food you like. Now, imagine the food you like is mixed in with the food you

hate. Imagine eating the two foods together, the food you love and the food you hate. Keep imagining the taste and texture of the two together. Keep eating them in your mind, a big plate, swallow them down, as you squeeze your thumb and little finger together. That's it, eat even more, more, and more until you can't eat any more, then stop.

6. Think about the food you used to like and notice how it's different now.

You can repeat this process as often as you like until you have completely eliminated your desire for that particular food. You will no longer be a slave to your cravings.

FREQUENTLY ASKED QUESTIONS ABOUT
"Craving Busters"

Q. What if I drink a lot?
Can I still lose weight?

Let's get really honest here—you're not fat because of what you drink. After all, there are plenty of thin alcoholics. The real issue with excessive drinking isn't weight gain, it's unconsciousness—and I'm not talking about drinking until you pass out!

Most people drink so that they don't have to deal with what's really going on in their lives—but now that you've begun this program, what's really going on in your life is a process of continual, positive change. I would suggest that at least at first, don't drink when you eat and don't eat when you are drinking, but if you do, just make sure to continue to follow the four golden rules of the system.

If you think you have a drinking problem, then seek help from an appropriate professional.

Q. I was doing really well but then I had a binge over the weekend—is it worth carrying on or should I wait until I've got my life more under control?

Your life will never be under control until you begin to control yourself—and every one of the tools in this system will help you. Following the four golden rules, learning to manage your emotions, and moving your body are all disciplines—but they get easier and easier the more you do them. In addition, the more control you gain over your eating, the more positive benefits you'll begin to experience in other areas of your life. It's not uncommon for people to report less stress, greater happiness, and even increased income as a result of applying this system over time.

As for the binge, forgive yourself and move on. It's not unusual and it's not your fault. As some of the old patterns of overeating dissipate, cravings arise. But now that you have the tools from this chapter, you'll be able to tap, tap, tap them away!

7

The Final Piece of the Weight-Loss Puzzle

Stopping Self-Sabotage Before It Starts

Remember, if you want to lose weight and keep it off for life, all you have to do is:

1. Eat when you're hungry.

2. Eat what you want, not what you think you should eat.

3. Enjoy every mouthful.

4. Stop when you think you might be full.

So what could possibly stop you from following these four simple principles?

I worked with a woman at one of our one-day weight-loss events whom I'll call Sheila. She had read the book, listened to the CD, and actually lost more than ten pounds in the first six weeks of working with the system. But then, as she put it, "life intervened." A crisis came up in her relationship with her daughter, her car stopped running, and she had a series of minor illnesses over the course of the next few months.

"The system," she said, "stopped working."

While I felt some empathy for her problems, I knew that what she really needed to hear was this:

Life will always intervene, and there will always be things that are clamoring for your attention. But if you really want to lose weight, increase your confidence, and feel great inside, you have to remember that you are in charge of you.

Regardless of what is going on in your life right now, you are the only one opening your mouth and shoving food into it when you're not really hungry, and you are the one letting your mind pay attention to everything but the delightful sensations and flavors of your breakfast, lunch, and dinner.

The system never stops working—
you stop following it.

And the good news is, you can restart your weight loss right now by simply tuning in to your body, noticing where you are on the Hunger Scale, and following the four golden rules day by day.

To my delight, Sheila came back for another course six months later, forty-two pounds lighter but, far more important, glowing from the inside out with a sense of achievement and new possibility.

When I talked to the 29 percent of people who couldn't get the system to work for them, it always came down to the same thing: they weren't following the system.

Sometimes, it was an active distrust:

- "I thought you were going to make me stop eating cream cakes and I love them."

- "He can't really mean eat *whenever* you're hungry—I'll just use the system during my one meal a day."

- "I'm sure he didn't mean eat what you *actually* want all the time—surely he just wants us to treat ourselves from time to time. I'll stick with the baked skinless chicken breasts but I'll have a bit of whipped cream on my low-fat no-sugar-added diet cardboard cake."

- "Dieting's not that bad—after all, I lost weight before my wedding by starving myself. I'll just use this as a set of guidelines for making my diet work better."

If any of this sounds like you, the choice is simple: follow my system *completely* and lose weight easily, or throw this book on the pile with the other failed diet manuals. I don't know any psychological system or drug that works for everyone all the time, but I can absolutely guarantee you that it won't work if you don't follow it.

But what was really interesting to me were the people who didn't even realize they weren't following the system. Consciously, they were completely engaged and committed, but unconsciously they were carrying hidden beliefs that were sabotaging their success.

Many people who hear this idea immediately recognize that it's true for them, but don't know what to do about it. Others ask, "But if my self-sabotage beliefs are unconscious, how can I know what they are?"

The good news is: you don't have to know what your unconscious beliefs are in order to change them.

Creating Wholeness

Have you ever heard people talk about "a part" of themselves? For example, they might say, "A part of me wants to go to the movies, but part of me wants to stay at home," or, "Part of me wants to get my work done but part of me wants to goof off for the day."

It's not as though there are actually "parts" inside you. It's simply different aspects of your consciousness that are temporarily in conflict. And when two or more "parts" of you are butting heads, the one that's strongest at that time will determine your behavior and the eventual outcome.

Sometimes you will hear it as "I want to ask that person out, but I am afraid I'll get rejected" or "I feel torn—I know what I need to do but I can't bring myself to do it." So one part of them wants to take action or to be in a relationship and another part is trying to protect against the pain of rejection.

What about you? Is there a part of you that really wants to lose weight, but another part that's not so sure? Do you find yourself firmly resolving that this time you're really going to do it, only to go unconscious and return to trying to satisfy your emotional hunger with french fries?

When this happens, it's a bit like driving down the street with one foot on the accelerator and the other on the brake: you may make progress, but you won't enjoy the journey and neither will anyone around you.

Over the years I have heard a vast array of reasons for self-sabotage of my system and even though they may not be logical, they serve an important purpose for the person who thinks them:

- "I have failed so many times in the past, I am worried that I will lose weight, but then put it all back on and feel really disappointed."

- "I had an affair because I was attractive and nearly lost my marriage. I am worried that if I lose weight it will happen again."

- "This is so simple it's too good to be true. I have spent years trying to lose weight and it's been very difficult. I will be furious with myself if this works for all the time and effort I have wasted."

- "I was abused and it was because I was beautiful and thin; I am frightened to lose weight in case it happens again."

Even though these may not sound like very logical reasons to stay overweight, they make perfect sense to anyone who understands how the unconscious really works. Your unconscious mind is not logical, it's purposeful—and its primary purpose is to ensure your survival and safety, no matter what the price.

This is the most important thing for you to know:

Every part of you has a positive intention.

The part that wants to lose weight wants you to feel good about yourself and be healthy. The part that's worried you'll fail and feel disappointed is trying to protect you from feelings of unhappiness. Even though they are taking you in seemingly opposite directions, they both share the same overriding intention: they both want the best for you. And when you apply the technique I am about to share with you, they will begin to work together for your highest good.

Creating Integrated Self-Belief

1. Identify the two conflicting beliefs or positions within your mind. For example, part of you may want to lose weight, but another part of you may want to stay overweight because it believes that will keep you safe. Or maybe you are scared you will fail and feel upset, so you might as well sabotage your attempts now and get it over with.

2. Place your hands out in front of you, palms up. Imagine the part that wants to lose weight in your right hand and the "sabotage" part in your left.

3. Ask each part in turn what its positive intention for you is in wanting what it wants. Continue asking until you really recognize that at some level they both want the same thing. Even if it feels like you are just making it up, going through this process will create dramatic changes in your levels of confidence and self-belief.

   Example:

   Weight loss ➤ more attractive ➤ better health ➤ SUCCESS!

   Sabotage ➤ more cautious ➤ feel safe ➤ SUCCESS!

4. Imagine a new, "super part" in between your hands with the combined resources of both your weight loss and your sabotage. So, for example, can you lose weight in a way in which you feel safe?

WEIGHT LOSS   SABOTAGE

5. Moving only as quickly as you can, bring your hands together until the two separate parts become one with the super part.

WEIGHT LOSS SABOTAGE **SUPER PART**

6. Bring your hands in to your chest and take the new integrated image inside you.

As you practice this technique, you will find it becomes easier and easier to resolve every internal conflict in this way. And when all parts of yourself are aligned and moving in the same direction, you will have become focused like a laser beam on whatever you decide to do!

(This technique used with the written permission of Dr. Richard Bandler)

FREQUENTLY ASKED QUESTIONS ABOUT

"The Final Piece of the Weight-Loss Puzzle"

Q. It's been nearly a week and I haven't lost any weight yet. What am I doing wrong?

Do you mean besides the fact that you're weighing yourself before the first two weeks are up?

There's an old story about a farmer who gave his daughter a package of seeds to plant so that she would learn about the natural order of planting and nurturing what you most want to see develop and grow. Yet even though he had given her some of the simplest growing seeds available, nothing new ever seemed to emerge from the field.

One day, the farmer noticed his daughter digging up the seeds and holding them up to the light. When he asked her what she was doing, she told him she wanted to see if there was anything growing yet. What she didn't realize was that each time she dug up a seed, she was preventing it from evolving at its natural pace.

In the same way, if you keep weighing yourself without allowing time for these seeds to take root in your unconscious, the only things that will grow are your stomach, hips, and thighs.

Q. What do I do if I fall off the wagon?

It's perfectly okay to make mistakes. As a baby, did you walk on your first attempt? When you learned to ride a bike, did you wobble at first and fall off a few times? Have the world's greatest achievers made mistakes on their journeys to success?

I would assume that in the first few weeks it's highly likely you will slip and overeat, or temporarily forget to follow the rules. It's fine—just return to following the rules again. Some people use a little slip to beat themselves up and tell themselves that once again they have failed; they console themselves with a binge or just give up on the system, resigned to the fact that they will always be fat.

Not this time! Simply go back to following the rules, eat when you are hungry, enjoy each mouthful, and when you suspect you are full, stop!

Q. I started losing weight, but now it's stopped. What do I do?

1. Are you eating whenever you're hungry?

2. Are you eating what you actually want, not what you think you should?

3. Are you eating consciously and enjoying every mouthful?

4. Are you stopping when you think you're full (even if there's still food on your plate)?

If you can honestly answer yes to each of these questions, then the secret is to *slow your eating speed down even more!*

Here's how it works: your stomach expands and contracts according to how much food you put into it. In the past, you were eating so fast you couldn't hear your body's "full" signal. Consequently, you overate and expanded your stomach, thereby creating a need for more food to make you full. When you began to slow down your eating speed, you became conscious of what you were eating as you were eating it and were able to notice the full signal much more quickly. You ate less food, your stomach contracted, and you needed less and less food to become full.

However, our bodies are highly adaptive. By now, you may have become so used to eating at your new, slower speed that you have once again become unconscious of what's going on with your body as you eat. By slowing down even more, you will once again "trick yourself awake," and be able to once again tune in to your body's satiation signals.

A Final Note

We are at the end of the book—and the beginning of a life in which you are in control of your body and what you do (and don't!) put in it.

Everything else in this book is here to help—and it will. You don't have to believe it, just follow my instructions.

Need some extra motivation? Review chapter 3 and spend some time seeing yourself slim.

Finding yourself in an eating frenzy? Review the information in chapter 4 on emotional eating or, if it's more urgent, go straight to the Craving Busters and tap your troubles away.

Perhaps the most important resource you have is the hypnosis CD, which I have created to assist you in making what used to be difficult changes easy and enjoyable. Listen to it every day to reinforce the positive changes you have already begun to make.

Remember, I can make you thin—but it's up to you to take the simple daily actions that will make being thin a habit—and some habits were made to last a lifetime!

Until we meet,

—Paul McKenna

How to Use the Success Journal

The weight-loss system you are about to embark upon is the most successful in the world. If it were a pill, I could sell it to a drug company for a billion dollars. But it's not a pill, it's a system—a system so simple that, at first, most people can't believe it will work for them.

The best thing is, you don't have to believe in it and there's no willpower required. All you have to do is just follow my instructions, and your life will dramatically change for the better.

According to the American Society of Training and Development, the likelihood of your doing something if you agree to check in with someone for accountability rises from only 40 percent to a whopping 95 percent!

So put simply: what gets measured gets done. Many people are now beginning to appreciate the power of journaling. Just keeping a simple daily log makes a significant difference in keeping you on track. A sample week's journal follows.

Over the next seven days, as you check the boxes and make a few simple notes about your progress, you will reinforce new habits that will change you relationship with food forever.

Day 1: Today's Success Checklist

		Check	Comments
1	I ate when I was hungry	☐	_____
2	I ate what I *really* wanted	☐	_____
3	I ate consciously	☐	_____
4	I stopped when full	☐	_____
5	I drank water	☐	_____
6	I moved my body	☐	_____
7	I listened to the CD	☐	_____
8	I did the mirror exercise	☐	_____

One **POSITIVE THING** I noticed today . . .

_____

_____

_____

What I'm **LOOKING FORWARD TO** tomorrow . . .

_____

_____

_____

Day 2: Today's Success Checklist

		Check	Comments
1	I ate when I was hungry	☐	_____
2	I ate what I *really* wanted	☐	_____
3	I ate consciously	☐	_____
4	I stopped when full	☐	_____
5	I drank water	☐	_____
6	I moved my body	☐	_____
7	I listened to the CD	☐	_____
8	I did the mirror exercise	☐	_____

One **POSITIVE THING** I noticed today . . .

_____

_____

_____

What I'm **LOOKING FORWARD TO** tomorrow . . .

_____

_____

_____

Day 3: Today's Success Checklist

		Check	Comments
1	I ate when I was hungry	☐	_____
2	I ate what I *really* wanted	☐	_____
3	I ate consciously	☐	_____
4	I stopped when full	☐	_____
5	I drank water	☐	_____
6	I moved my body	☐	_____
7	I listened to the CD	☐	_____
8	I did the mirror exercise	☐	_____

One **POSITIVE THING** I noticed today . . .

_____

_____

_____

What I'm **LOOKING FORWARD TO** tomorrow . . .

_____

_____

_____

Day 4: Today's Success Checklist

		Check	Comments
1	I ate when I was hungry	☐	_____
2	I ate what I *really* wanted	☐	_____
3	I ate consciously	☐	_____
4	I stopped when full	☐	_____
5	I drank water	☐	_____
6	I moved my body	☐	_____
7	I listened to the CD	☐	_____
8	I did the mirror exercise	☐	_____

One **POSITIVE THING** I noticed today . . .

_____

_____

_____

What I'm **LOOKING FORWARD TO** tomorrow . . .

_____

_____

_____

Day 5: Today's Success Checklist

		Check	Comments
1	I ate when I was hungry	☐	_____
2	I ate what I *really* wanted	☐	_____
3	I ate consciously	☐	_____
4	I stopped when full	☐	_____
5	I drank water	☐	_____
6	I moved my body	☐	_____
7	I listened to the CD	☐	_____
8	I did the mirror exercise	☐	_____

One **POSITIVE THING** I noticed today . . .

_____

_____

_____

What I'm **LOOKING FORWARD TO** tomorrow . . .

_____

_____

_____

Day 6: Today's Success Checklist

		Check	Comments
1	I ate when I was hungry	☐	_____
2	I ate what I *really* wanted	☐	_____
3	I ate consciously	☐	_____
4	I stopped when full	☐	_____
5	I drank water	☐	_____
6	I moved my body	☐	_____
7	I listened to the CD	☐	_____
8	I did the mirror exercise	☐	_____

One **POSITIVE THING** I noticed today . . .

_____

_____

_____

What I'm **LOOKING FORWARD TO** tomorrow . . .

_____

_____

_____

Day 7: Today's Success Checklist

		Check	Comments
1	I ate when I was hungry	☐	_____
2	I ate what I *really* wanted	☐	_____
3	I ate consciously	☐	_____
4	I stopped when full	☐	_____
5	I drank water	☐	_____
6	I moved my body	☐	_____
7	I listened to the CD	☐	_____
8	I did the mirror exercise	☐	_____

One **POSITIVE THING** I noticed today . . .

_____

_____

_____

What I'm **LOOKING FORWARD TO** tomorrow . . .

_____

_____

_____

Index of Techniques

Index

Index

About the Author

PAUL McKENNA, PhD, is the "Dr. Phil" of Britain. He is the United Kingdom's best-selling nonfiction author, having sold 3 million books in the last three years. He has worked with Hollywood movie stars, Olympic gold medalists, rock stars, top business achievers, and royalty. The *Times of London* recently named McKenna one of the world's leading and most important modern self-help gurus. For years, Paul McKenna has helped millions of people successfully quit smoking, lose weight, overcome insomnia, eliminate stress, and increase self-confidence.

In the spring of 2008 he had a hit TV series on TLC called *I Can Make You Thin*. This unique interactive program has already been a massive success in the UK and McKenna's system has changed the way millions of people lose weight in Europe. Now he's coming to America!

Would you like to work with Paul McKenna as your personal weight loss coach?

How much more successful do you think you could be in reaching your goals?

As an additional resource for readers of this book, Paul has now created a membership web site at **www.mckenna.com** where you can get complete support in reaching your weight loss goals.

- A 14-day jumpstart program customized to your personal weight loss needs

- Members-only access to Paul's regular podcast where you can call and talk with him directly about your personal weight loss issues

- Access to an online library of video and audio clips, including mini-movies of Paul demonstrating every technique in this book

- A unique online 90-day success journal to guide you through the crucial first three months of applying the system

- Daily tips and exclusive advice from bestselling author and life coach to the Hollywood elite Michael Neill demonstrating every technique in this book

- A sense of belonging, camaraderie, and friendship with other members of one of the largest online weight loss communities in the world!

To join the club and learn more, visit
www.mckenna.com